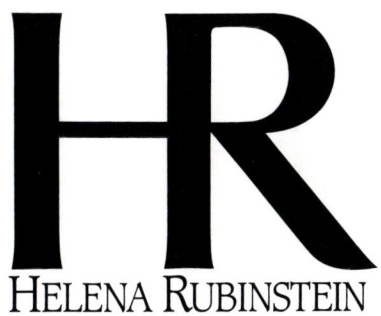

© 2002 Assouline Publishing for the present edition
601 West 26th Street, 18th floor
New York, NY 10001, USA
Tel.: 212 989-6810   Fax: 212 647-0005
www.assouline.com

First published by Editions Assouline, Paris, France

Color separation: Gravor (Switzerland)
Printed by Grafiche Milani (Italy)

ISBN: 2 84323 426 3

All rights reserved.
No part of this publication may be reproduced, stored in a retrieval system,
or transmitted in any form or by any means, electronic, mechanical,
photocopying, recording, or otherwise, without prior consent from the publisher.

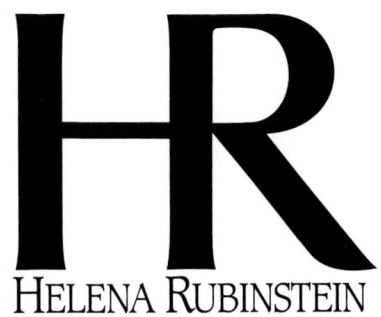

# HR
## Helena Rubinstein

**Catherine Jazdzewski**

**ASSOULINE**

Jean Cocteau called her the Empress of Beauty. Demanding, passionate, headstrong, inquisitive, authoritarian, and charming, Helena Rubinstein was an extraordinary personality who was capable of applying her keen business acumen to the emerging industry of cosmetology. She was a creative visionary, the first person to open a beauty salon, which she did at the beginning of the twentieth century, thus combining dermatology with cosmetics, and the inventor of skin creams which would later be emulated by the cosmetics industry worldwide. She was fascinated by all forms of beauty, painting and design and women's face. She looked at the latter closely, examined them as one would a painting, and did everything she could to make them more beautiful.

"A good story is always better than the truth", was one of her favourite sayings. "Never look back! There's no point. No one likes to remember the truth", so let's begin with the legend. Helena Rubinstein was born on 25 December 1872 in Cracow, a peaceful and devout city in Poland whose city walls surround one of the oldest universities in Europe, where the students read mathematics, classics and theolgy. Her father was a passionate collector of art and antiques, her mother a model of intuition and tenderness. The Rubinstein were a very loving family. There were another seven daughters — Pauline, Rosa, Regina, Stella, Ceska, Manka, and Erna. Yet, at the age of twenty, Helena Rubinstein left this affectionate and cultured atmosphere for the heat and dust of Australia. She hunted at a broken love affair, but the truth was probably a lot less romantic. "Life was not easy for Jews in Eastern Europe", she once confided briefly. "We were humble people of modest means. Since I was the eldest daughter and there were no sons, I knew I had to help the family. Australia was the only way out. I had to get away and lead my own life." This young girl was starting to take on the mantle of the breadwinner she would become, a woman who built an empire, a family business, which she ran with her sisters, her sons and nieces (her great rival, Elisabeth Arden called it "the Polish mafia").

Before that that could happen, however, Rubinstein needed enormous courage to face the solitary journey, the unfamiliar destination and the total change of life which lay ahead. At the turn of the century, Australia was an arid land which the British considered to be one huge prison-camp. The sun was burning, the wind was abrasive, the countryside stretched away into infinity, flat and uninteresting, dotted here and there with an eucalyptus tree. It gave people "the pip", it even drove them mad. Helena Rubinstein, arrived in early 1892 and stayed with her maternal uncle, Louis Silberfeld, who was a sheep-farmer at Corelaine, an isolated spot about a hundred kilometres from Melbourne. Her relationship with her uncle deteriorated fast and she became bored. "I hated Australia. It was hell. Heat, misery, ugliness. I didn't get on well with my relations. But, I was ambitious. I wanted to show the world and my family what I was capable of." So she offered her services to the little town pharmacist, mixing his oinments and medicinal herbs, avidly studying her pharmacopœa. The medicinal formulas fascinated her and sealed her fate. Since so many women praised her lovely complexion and wanted to try her miracle cream, she decided to sell it to them!

The cream she was using, which she called *Valaze*, had been created by two chemists, the Lykusky brothers, who were friends of the Rubinstein family. She wrote to them and in reply they sent her the formula, which she started to prepare immediately . Why did she give the name *Valaze* to this miracle cream which protected against the ravages of wind and sun? No special reason : "It sounded good" she said. Edward Titus, a journalist friend — they would marry in 1908 — wrote an article vaunting the merits of this beneficial cream, which started her on the road to success. As soon as the article appeared, Rubinstein received fifteen thousand orders accompanied by the same number of cheques. She mixed the cream by hand, put it into pots, stuck on the labels, and although she worked day and night she still did not manage to fulfill all the orders. Reinforcements arrived from Poland in the shape of Dr. Lykusky who took charge of the manufacturing.

In 1902, Helena decided to open a beauty parlour in Melbourne which she called *Valaze*; it consisted of three rooms with examination cubicles and treatment areas. Melbourne thus became the first city in the world to have a Beauty salon. Helena Rubinstein was there in person to offer advice and care, thus inventing a new occupation, that of beautician. this is where she taught women who were frightened of wrinkles of sagging skin, of ageing. In 1905, her sister Ceska came over to join her. Together, they earned a hundred thousand dollars a year. Sydney and Brisbane were clamouring for *Valaze* beauty parlours. But Helena Rubinstein had her doubts, she was not sure he had enough knowledge, so she handed over the reins of the business to Ceska and went back to Europe. For two years, she travelled through Austria and Germany visiting Vienna, Dresden, Berlin, Hambourg, consulting or helping the greatest dermatologists, biologists, and dieticians of the day. "I wanterd to learn everything there was to know about the skin and the art of treating imperferctions."

In 1908, Helena Rubinstein and Edward Titus settled in London. They had a son, then another son. They opened the second *Valaze* salon in Mayfair, in what had been Lord Salisbury's town house. It was a triumph! The British aristocraty flocked there. Within ten years the young Polish immigrants had become rich and famous and had adopted her unique style. She was sumptuously dressed, bedecked in numerous jewels, her shining black hair drawn back into a severe bun, her lips bright red and her dark observant eyes ringed with eyeliner. "It's making a splash that counts", she would say. At the age of thirty, Helena Rubinstein was incredibly beautiful, gentle but firm, bright and intelligent, and above all, very authoritarian. Yet, she always spoke in a soft and hesitant voice, giving her that special attraction which meant no one could refuse her anything. Although she was a triumph in London, she was determined to continue her conquests and she worked incessantly, spending hours in her "kitchens", as she always called her laboratories and later, her factories. She was the first to invent and classify the different types of skin: greasy, normal or dry. The *Valaze* cream was turned into a complete product range including day and night cream, a *Black Pomade*, the first facial mask to prevent acne, and astringent tonics and fresheners such as *Eau d'or, Eau verte, Eau qui pique*.

"London is an elegant city, but everything starts from Paris." Paris became, and remained, the city of the heart. She moved there in 1921 and opened another *Valaze* in the Faubourg-Saint-Honoré, leaving the London salon to be run by her sister Manka. In Paris, she continued to defend the need for skin and body care, including the use of hot-and-cold showers, electrolysis and new hydrotherapy treatment. Having tried a massage, Colette wrote: "For a woman, it's a sacred duty to be massaged. It is a prerequisite for a French women: how else can they hope to keep a lover?" Helena Rubinstein painted her model's faces and created the first lipstick in tubes, as well as the first face powder coloured to match the complexion. At the home of Misia Sert, she met Proust. "He asked me questions about make-up. Does a duchess use rouge? Do *demi-mondaines* blackened their eyes with khôl?" She was also introduced to Bonnard, Vuillard, Renoir. If Melbourne had made her rich, and London famous, in Paris, she would discover her next passion after beauty — art.
She posed for Helleu, Dufy, Van Dongen, Marie Laurencin, … She introduced Picasso to primitive art, and gave Dalí a taste for money. Although, she never owned a car, — "they lost half their value from the first kilometre" — she bought canvas after canvas without ever disputing the price with the artist. Helena Rubinstein

was an aesthete who accumulated paintings in the same way that she governed — matriarchally. She did not collect, she preferred to provide for artists and launch them to stardom. Throughout her life, she created various artistic foundations. Fascinated by everything beautiful, she had eclectic tastes. In Paris as in New York, each of her apartments was a museum. Her Park Avenue drawing room was a mixture of Victorian chairs, Chinese tables and Turkish lamps, all of them on an acid-green carpet designed by Joan Miró. The walls were completely covered with an extroardinary assortment of paintings. Matisse, Braque, Chagall, Derain, Gris, Rouault, Picasso, Dalí, Tchelitchev were all represented. At her home in Paris, on the Quai de Béthune, Modigliani, Bonnard and Miró jostled for space alongside six hundred and twenty-two sculptures from Benin. The furniture was Boulle, French Regency and Louis-Philippe and the walls were hung with yellow silk. To her detractors, whe would reply: "There is a link between an African mask, a piece of Romantic furniture and a painting by Matisse. It is mysterious and strong, essential — in an aesthetic sense — for happiness." This quest for beauty was the symbol of her internal quest, her constant search for perfection.

World war I took Helena Rubinstein and her family to America. Then, she discovered the suffragettes, came into competition with Elisabeth and Charles Revson (Revlon) and the American way of doing business. She started the firm of *Helena Rubinstein, Valaze products* in New York — others would follow in Chicago, Boston and San Francisco — and learn to adapt to the rules of capitalism. Her products needed to be sold in department stores throughout the country. She acquiesced, but also imposed her own rules. Each distributor had to go through six months scientific training and the saleswomen were also carefully trained. The Food and Drug Administration did not like her advertising, so she introduced strict controls and imposed ever-more rigorous manufacturing procedures. She turned cosmetics into industry. Beauty was no longer the prerogative of an elite but came within the reach of all women, whatever their social class. In 1923, her catalogue contained eighty care products and one hundred and sixty items of make-up, including *Reducing Preparation* and other slimming creams.

Helena Rubinstein combined her intuitive creativity with an extraordinary business acumen. Against all expectations, in 1928 and a few months before the Wall Street crash, she sold her company for eight million dollars. The whole of New York agreed that the operation was an incredible case of financial foresight. She denied it claiming that she had done so in order to save her marriage, to Edward Titus - they had separated by then. Yet, a year later, she wrote personally to hundreds of small investors, mainly women, explaining the banks weren't interested in women's problems and enlisting their help. For less that two million dollars, she succeeded in buying back her company making a net profit of six million dollars, thus becoming one of the richest women in the world.

Contrary to what might be believed, Edward Titus, whose real name was Edward Ameisen, was neither British nor American, but Polish, like Rubinstein. He changed his name upon arrival in Australia, a fugitive from the pogroms. Both an intellectual and a man of taste, he owned an art gallery and publishing house in the Montparnasse district of Paris in the 1930s and published books by D.H. Lawrence, Hemingway and Joyce. As a journalist, he did a great deal to make Helena Rubinstein's name, while through their relationship, he helped to shape her personality. For instance, it was he who had the idea of calling her "Madame", which became her nickname used by colleagues, employees and family alike. Titus was a brilliant public relations man and publicist. He wrote the first advertisements for Valaze and initiated Helena Rubinstein into the art of copywriting. It was he who suggested that famous artists such as Marie Laurencin, Dufy or Dalí be commissioned to design powder compacts and he asked writers such as Louise de Vilmorin, Marie Laure de Noailles and Colette to provide some memorable catchphrases. Although he was the great and sole love of Helena Rubinstein's life, she never quite managed to combine work and marital bliss. The couple divorced in 1936. Two years later, she married the Georgian Prince Atchill Gourielli. With this man of the world, whose greatest passion was bridge, she had the latitude she needed to devote herself to the business.

In post-war Paris, a tiny, vivacious woman used to take the metro every morning to go to work in a shop without electricity in the Faubourg-Saint-Honoré. She was the former Helena Rubinstein, now Princess Gourielli. Many of her family members had perished in the Holocaust, the Germans had stolen or destroyed all her property in Europe but although she wasn't seventy years of age and was a multimillionairess in the United States, she was determined to start afresh and so set to work with the same energy and determination as she had in Melbourne. Once again, she began formulating creams putting them into pots and selling them. The parisian women starved of beauty and beauty products through the war, responded enthusiastically. Sales began to soar. Only five years later, the Helena Rubinstein company was number one in Europe. She hired young chemists, ruled her headquarters with a matriarchal fist, discussed all her plans with an excitment that was catching and took all the decisions. Even if this tenacious woman no longer made her own creams, each product was the result of her precise observations. All were well ahead of their time, amazing in their modernity. In 1950, she created *Deep Cleanser*, the first product of its type. In 1954, she introduced *Lanolin Vitamin Formula*, the first vitamin enriched cream, then *Contour Lift film*, to firm and lift the skin of the face. Then in 1956, *Skin Dew* became the world's first moisturing cream and *Longlash* the first automatically refillable mascara. In 1959, she was invited to the American Fair in Moscow, as one of only two cosmetics firms (the other was Coty). She had won the bet she made with herself as a young girl, that of building an empire. In the late 1950s, the Helena Rubinstein brand name was represented throughout the world with more than fourteen factories, thousands of points of sale and about forty thousand employees.

When Patrick O'Higgins, her private secretary who stayed with her until her death, first met her, she was eighty years old, but looked less than half that age: the reason for her eternal youthfulness was her power of concentration and her vitality", he said. "The force of her personality was amazing but at the same time she could be strangely motherly." Work always fuelled her energy. He took her on trips — she travelled round the world — to visit the subsidiary companies and give lectures. In 1965, the year of her death, she was still monitoring the whole business personally. "I want the business to carry on for at least three hundred years", she used to say.

a woman of vision. Helena Rubinstein created a visionary brand name. The Helena Rubinstein company has never broken the rules which its creator formulated. These are what constitute her ethic. And since Helena Rubinstein developped her beauty care products as pioneering events in the science of cosmetology, each subsequent product launch represented another technological advance. It was a challenge to create *Power A, face sculptor* and *Force C*. These products represented the success of inhouse research and became the benchmarks for the fight against the ravages of time on the femal complexion. Helena Rubinstein also revolutionnised make-up, thanks to her palette of products and colours. Today, the brand which bears her name has initiated a new wave of creativity with blue lipstick and gold nail polish, which are greeted enthusiastically by the press before becoming the latest fashions. Here again, these colours could not exist without technological daring.

Helena Rubinstein introduced an even more important innovation in the 1950s, when she created a foundation for the promotion of the rights and well-being of women and their children, the developpement of their education and their access to learning and culture. She joined with UNESCO in creating the Helena Rubinstein Prize for Women and Knowledge, thus perpetuating her moral values. Indeed, through her life, Helena Rubinstein helped to invent the future of women.

Helena Rubinstein
126
valaze
produits
de
beauté

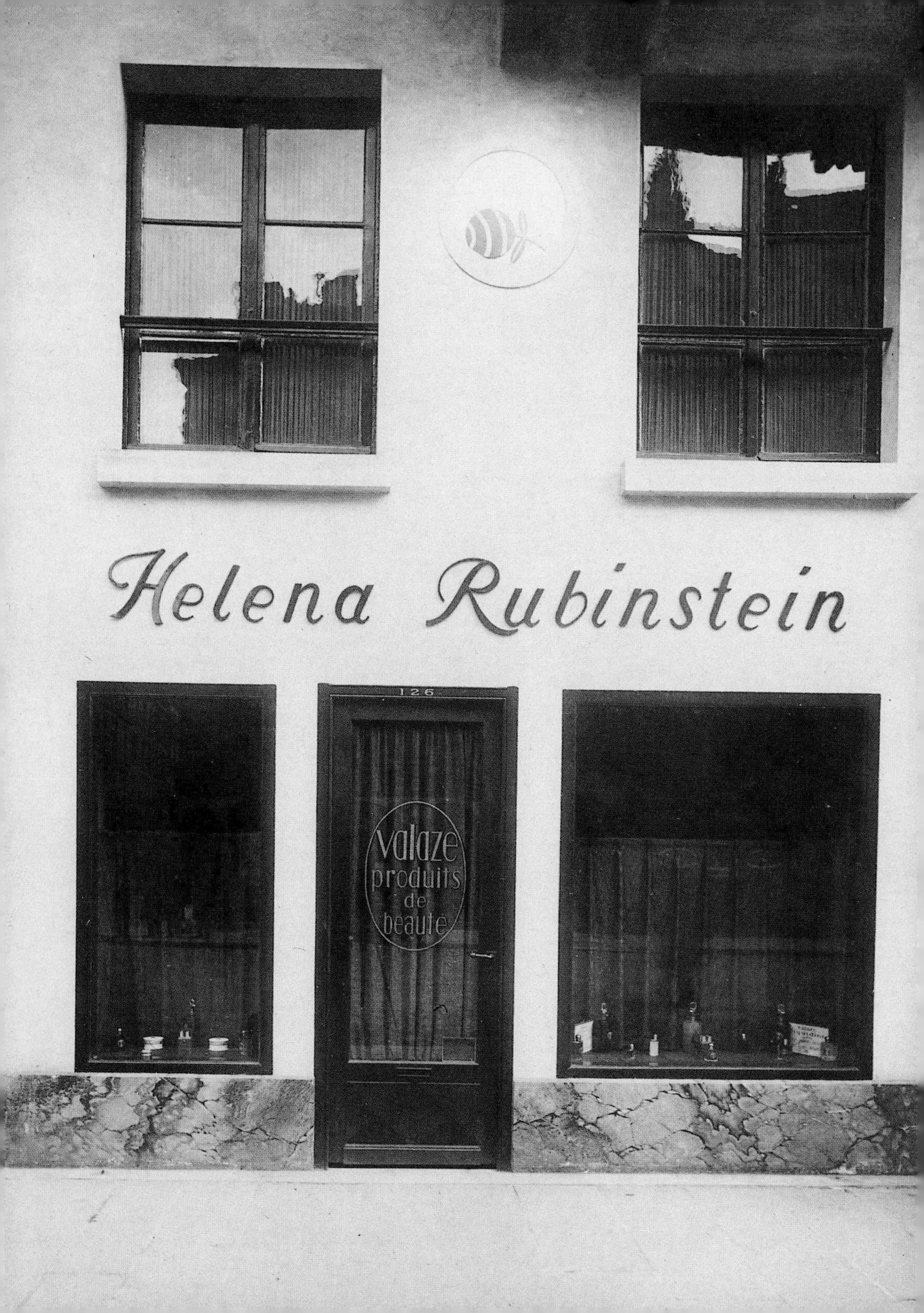

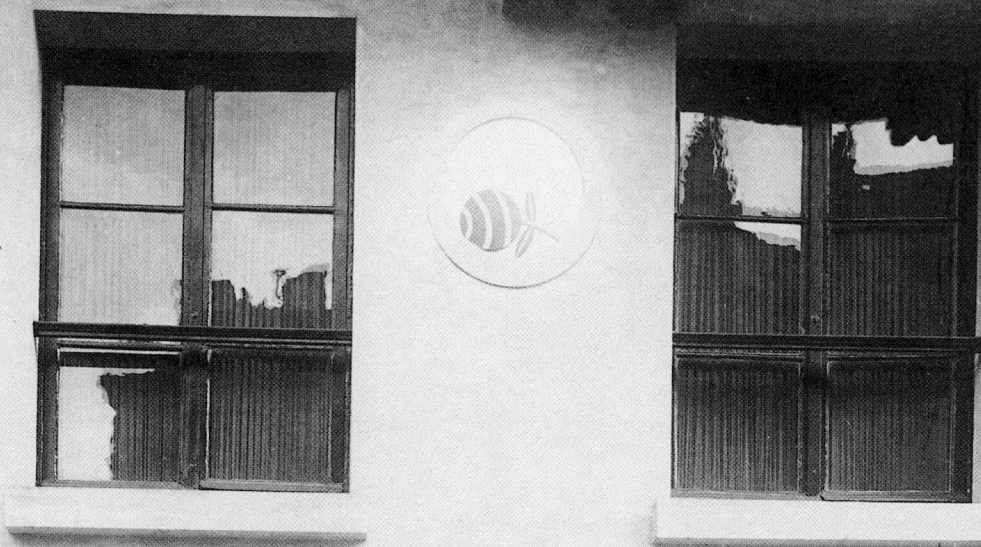

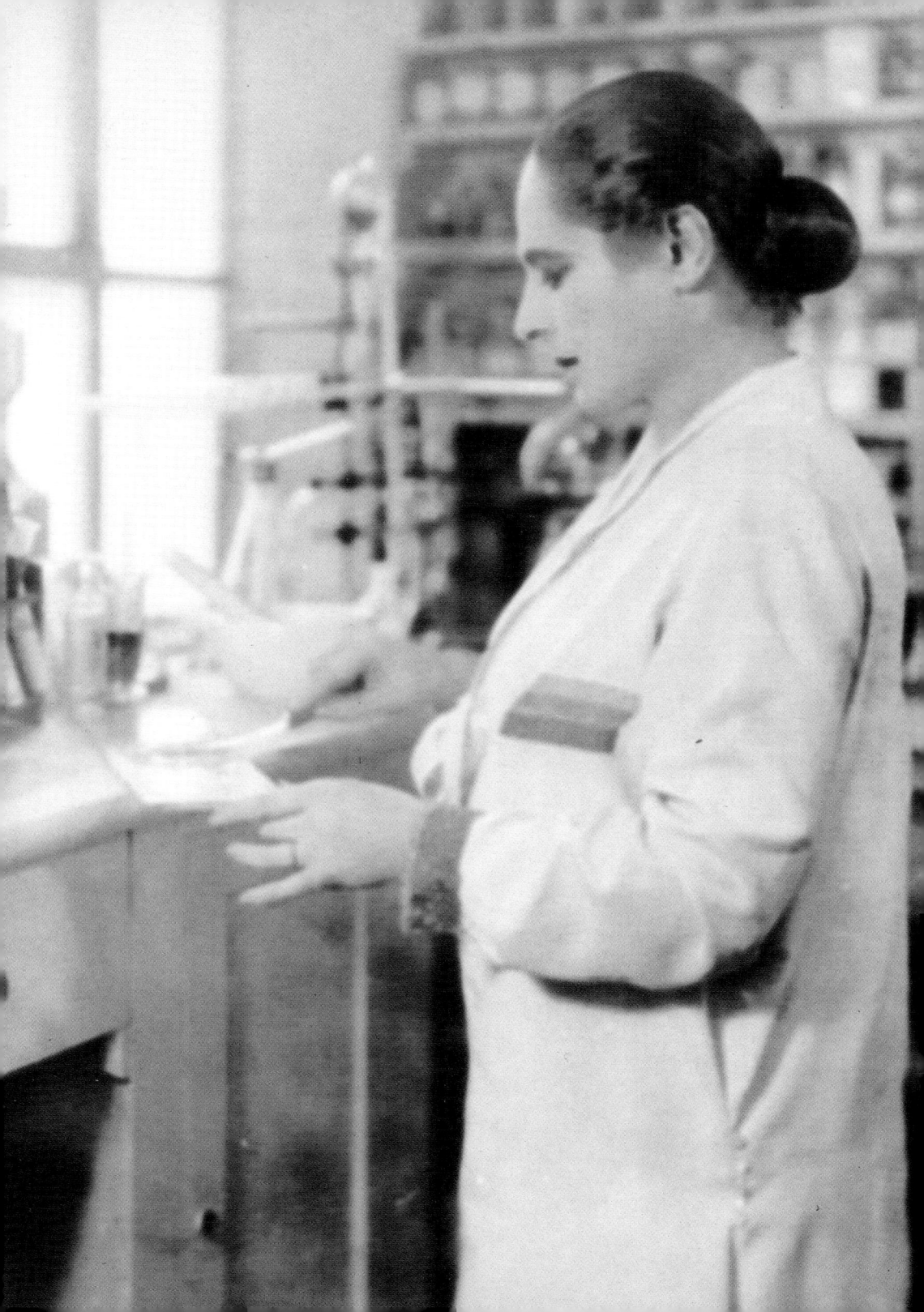

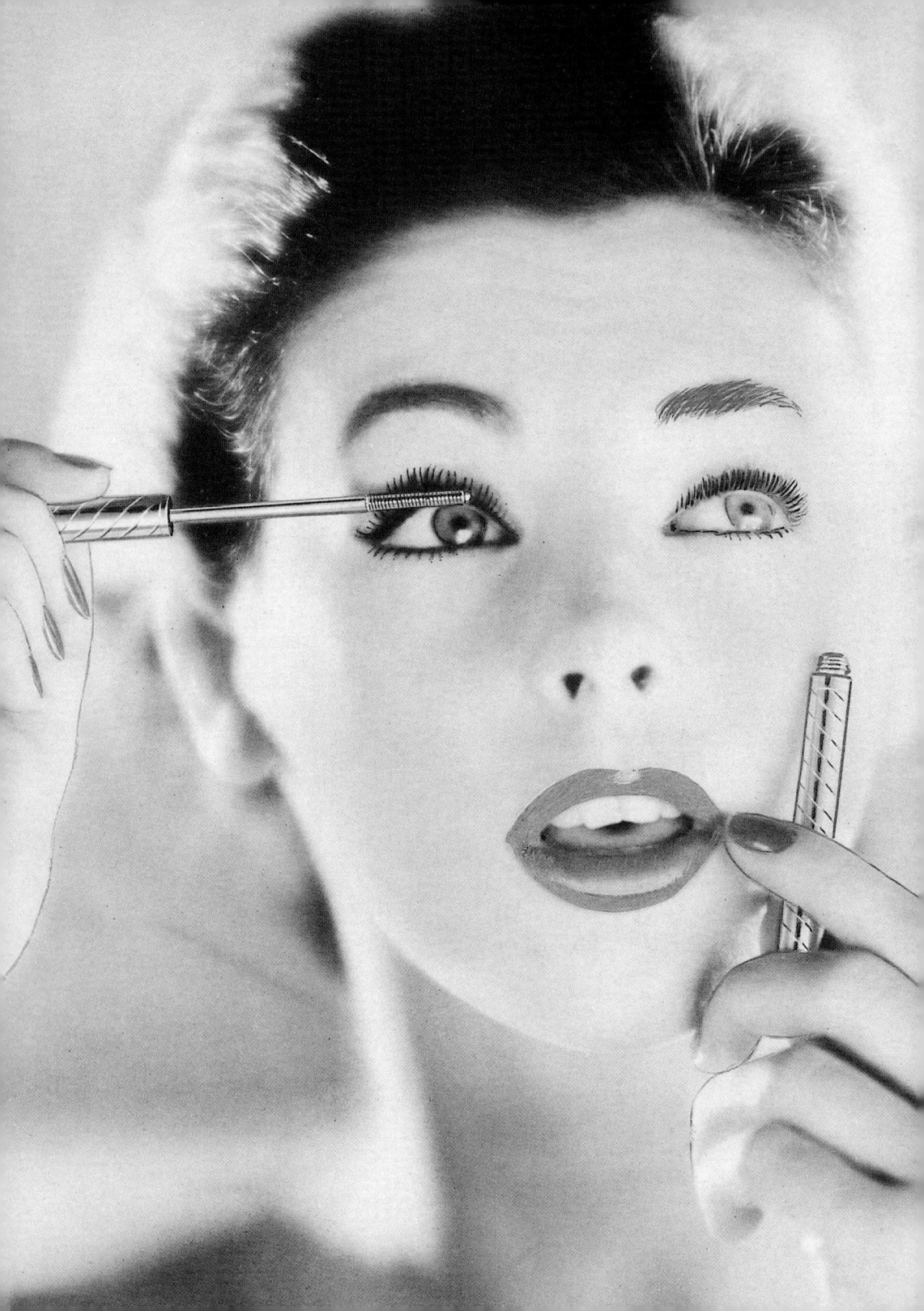

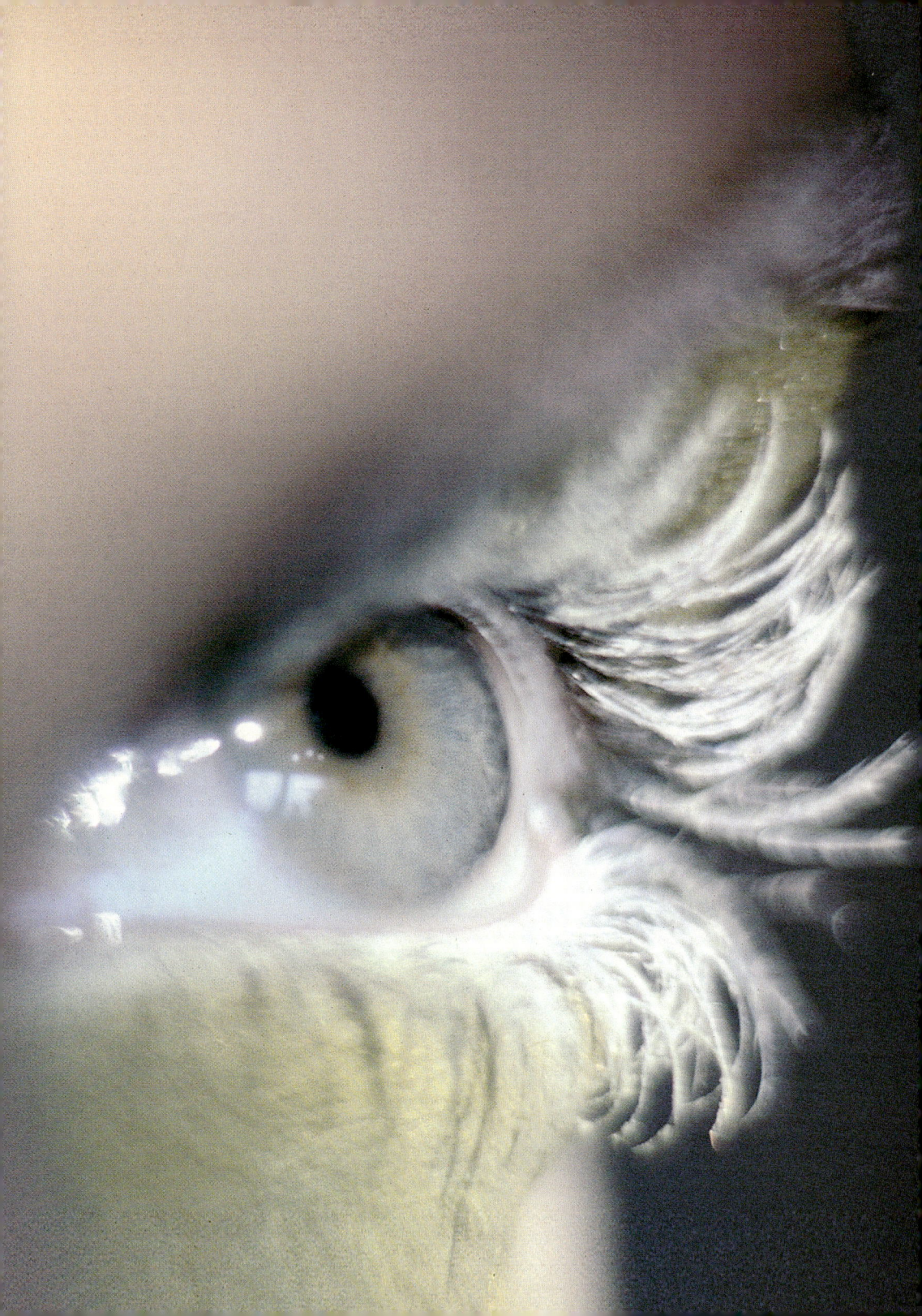

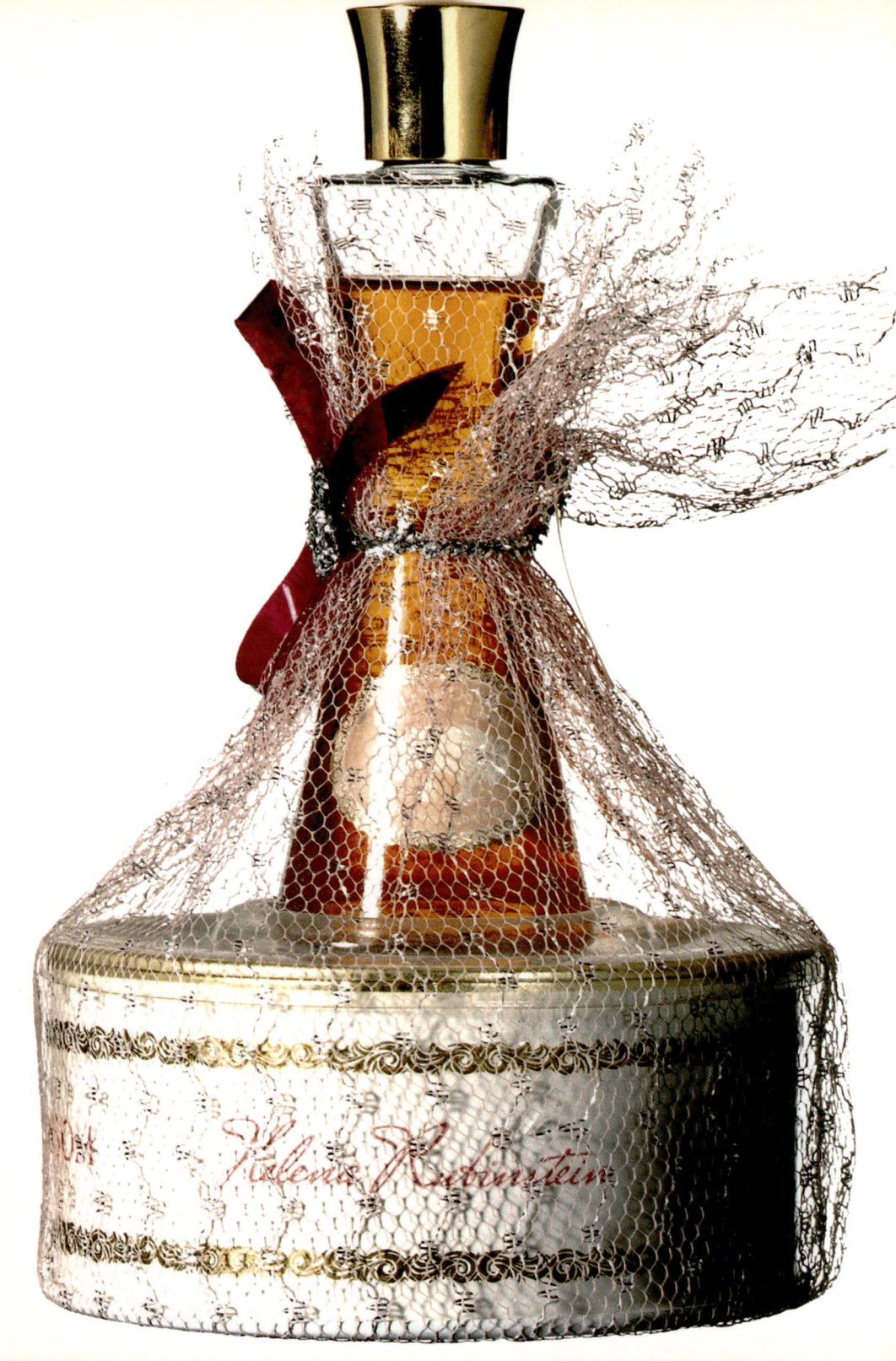

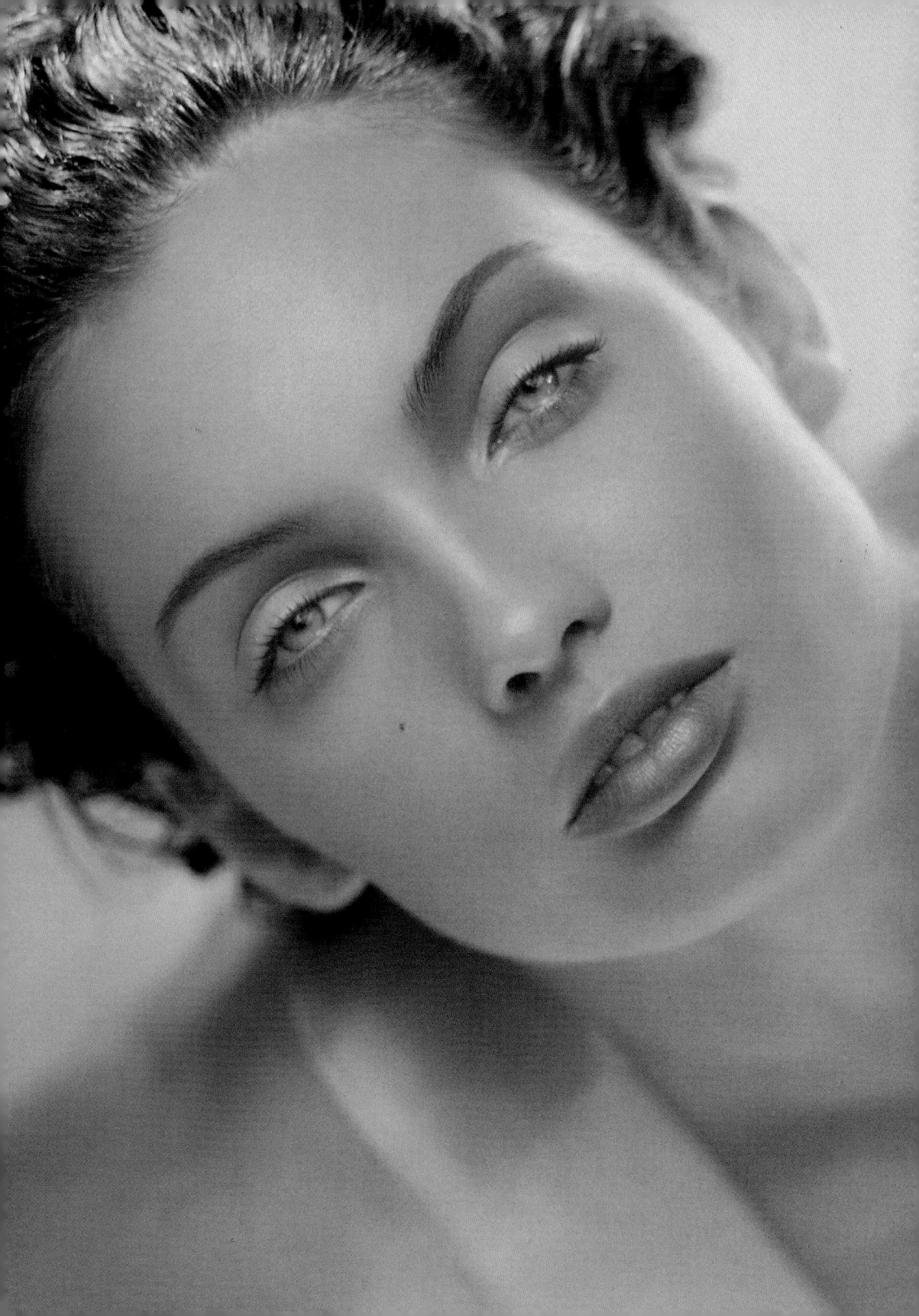

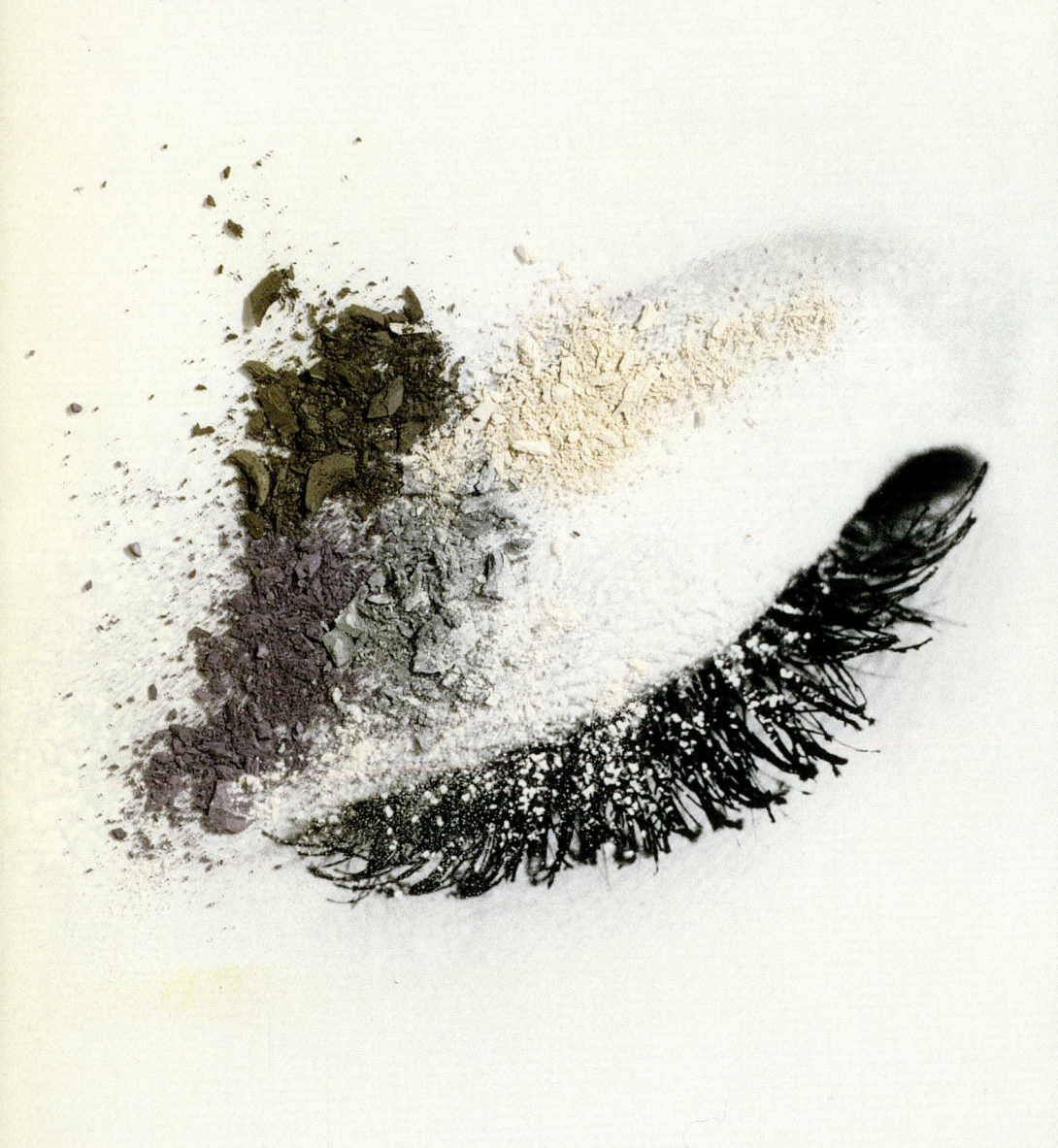

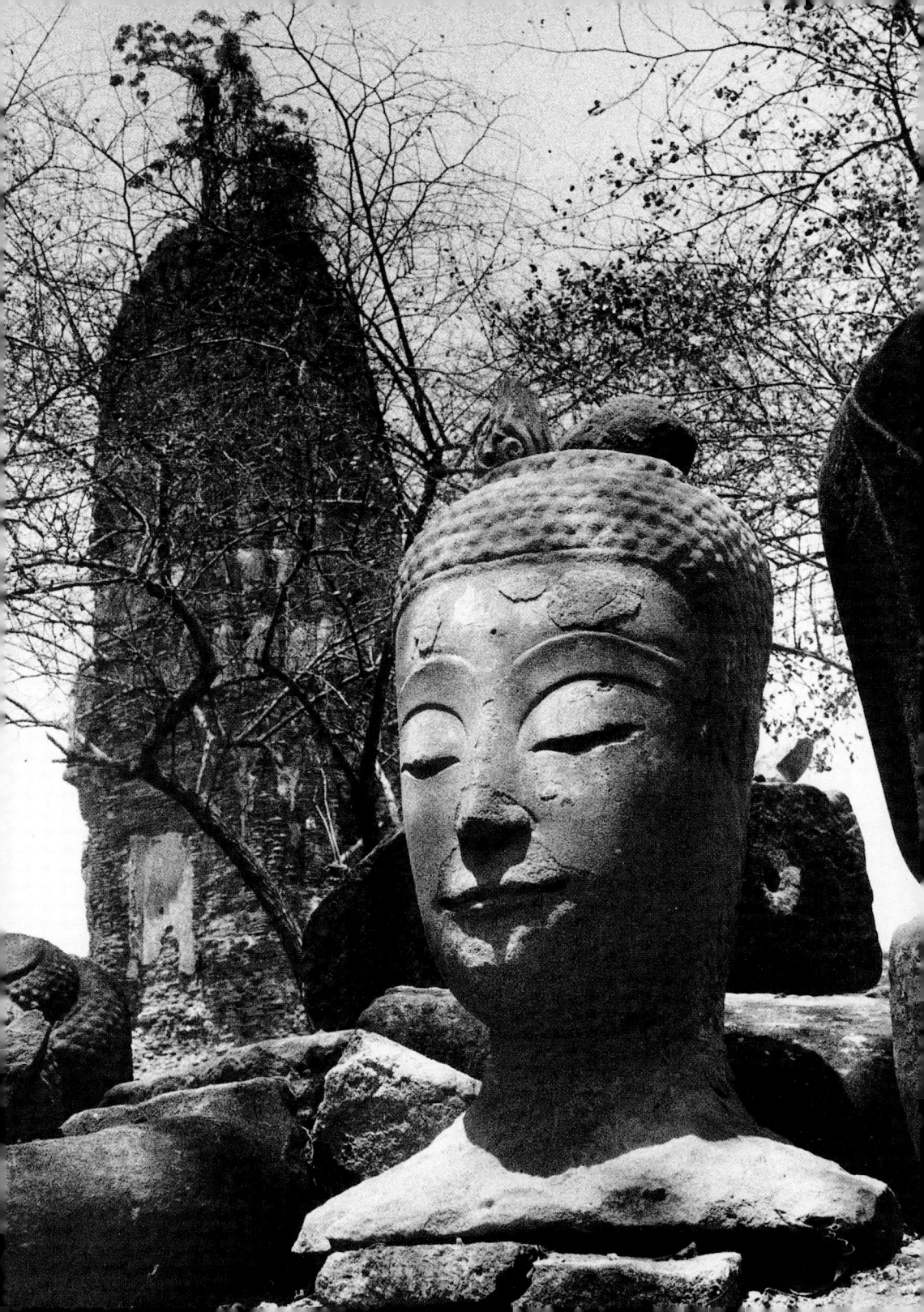

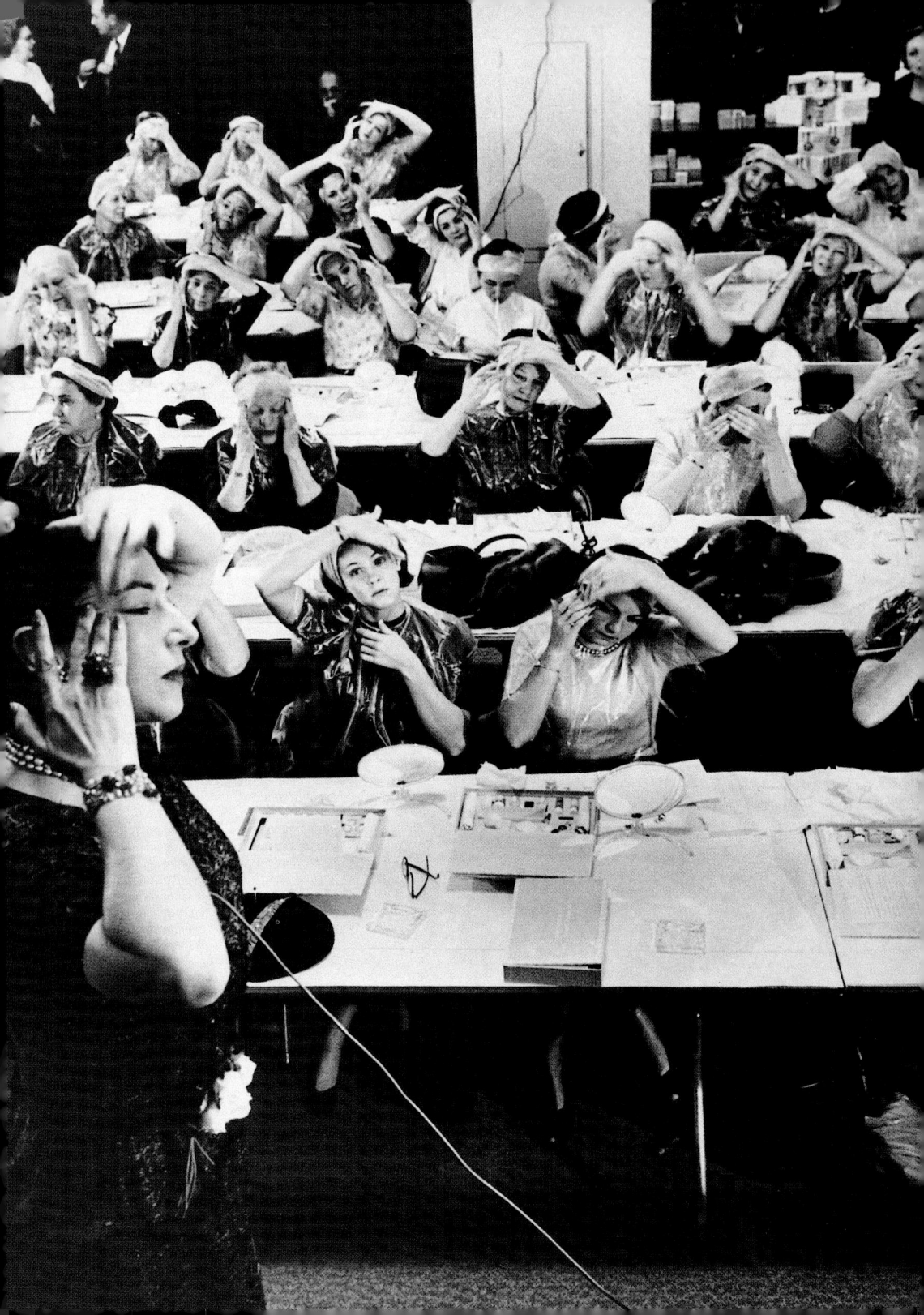

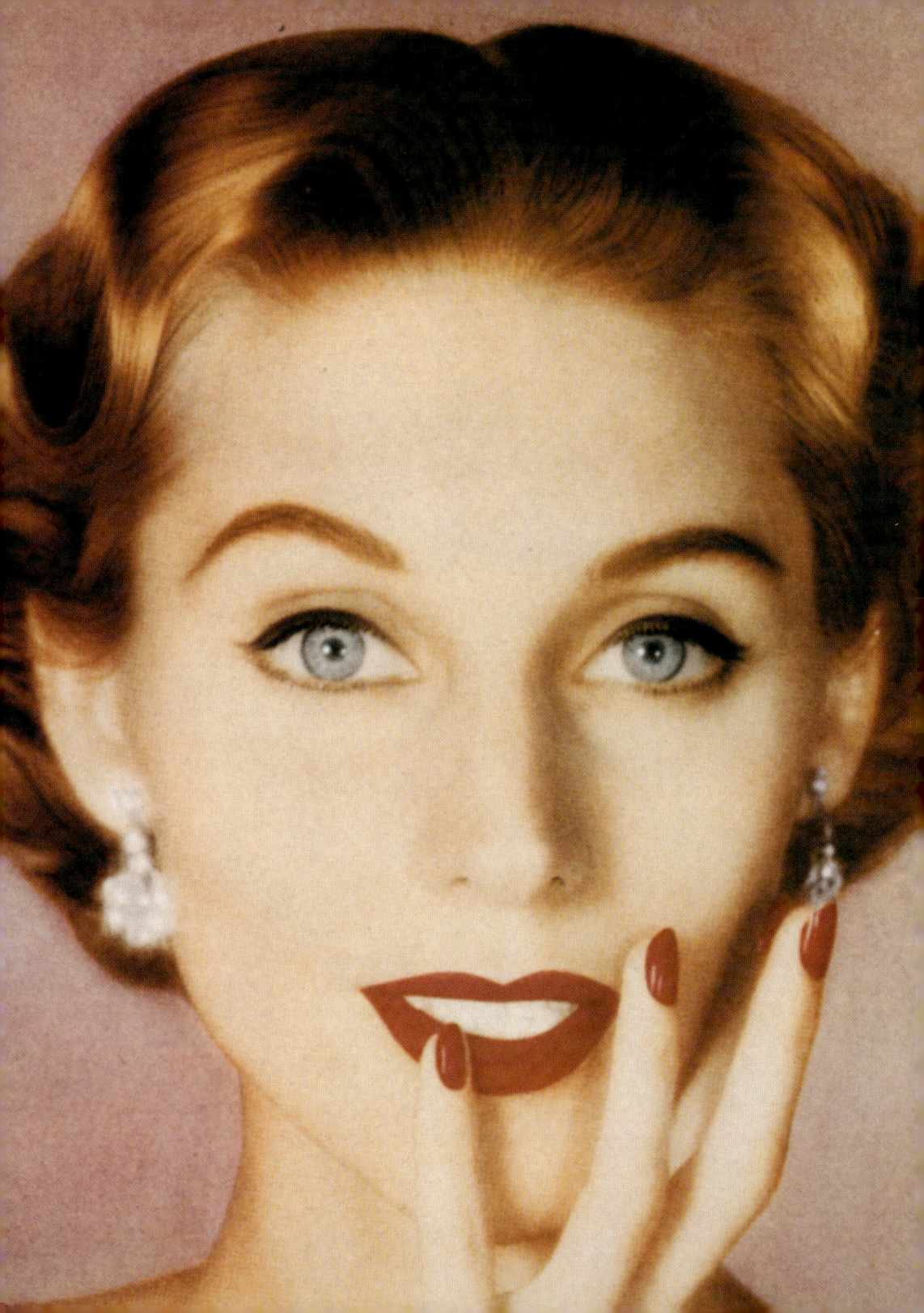

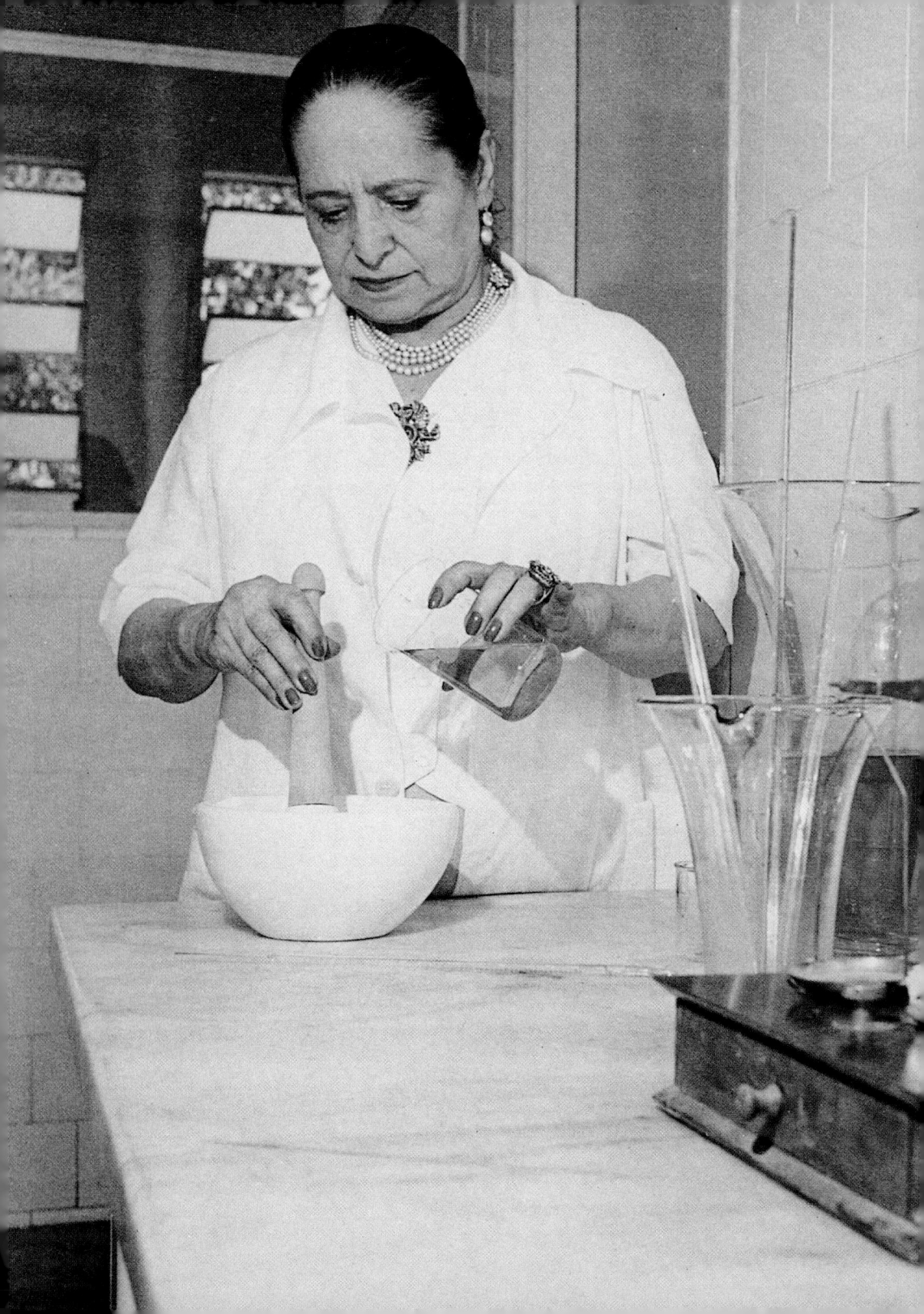

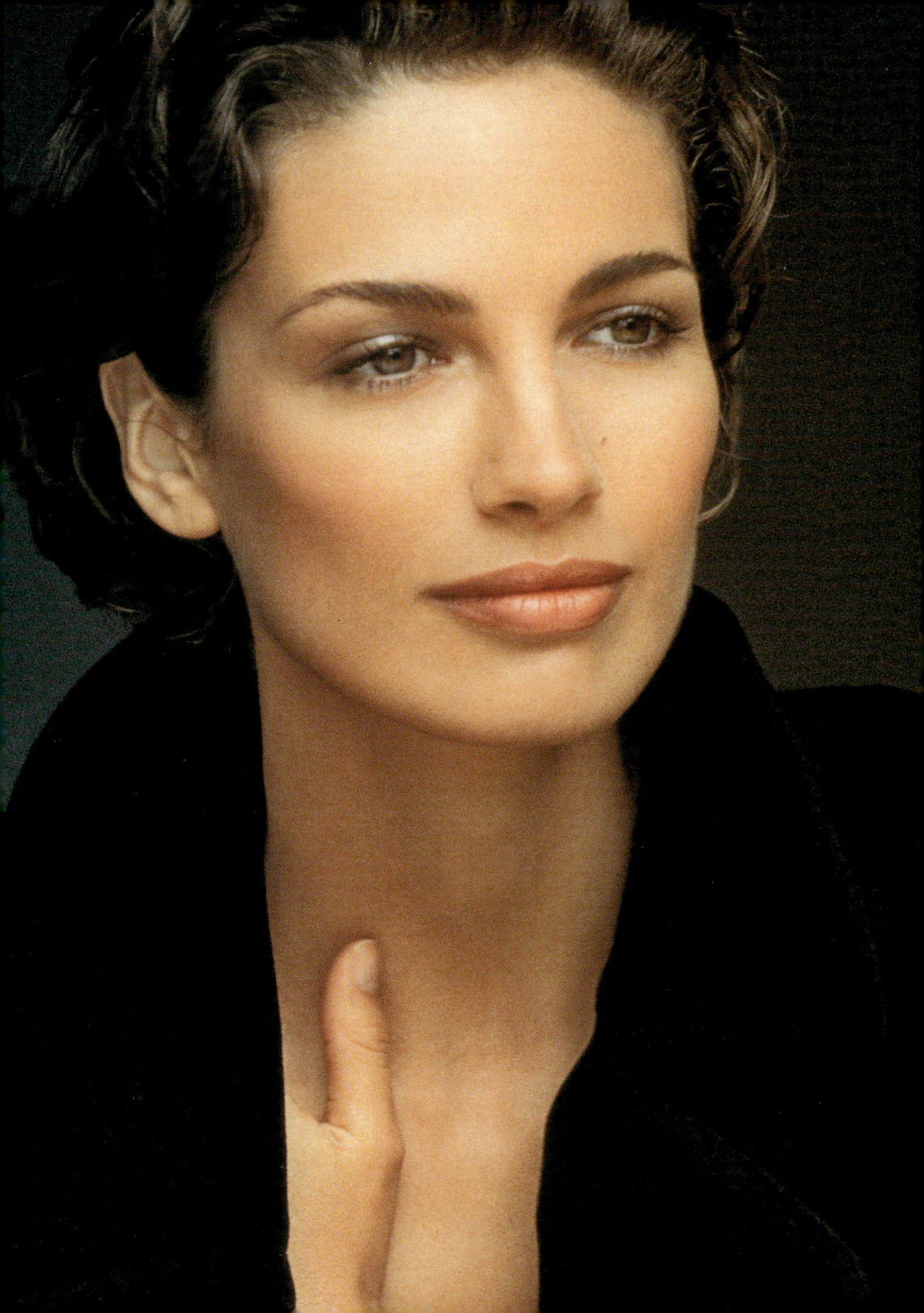

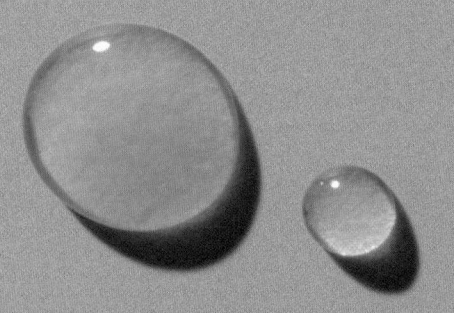

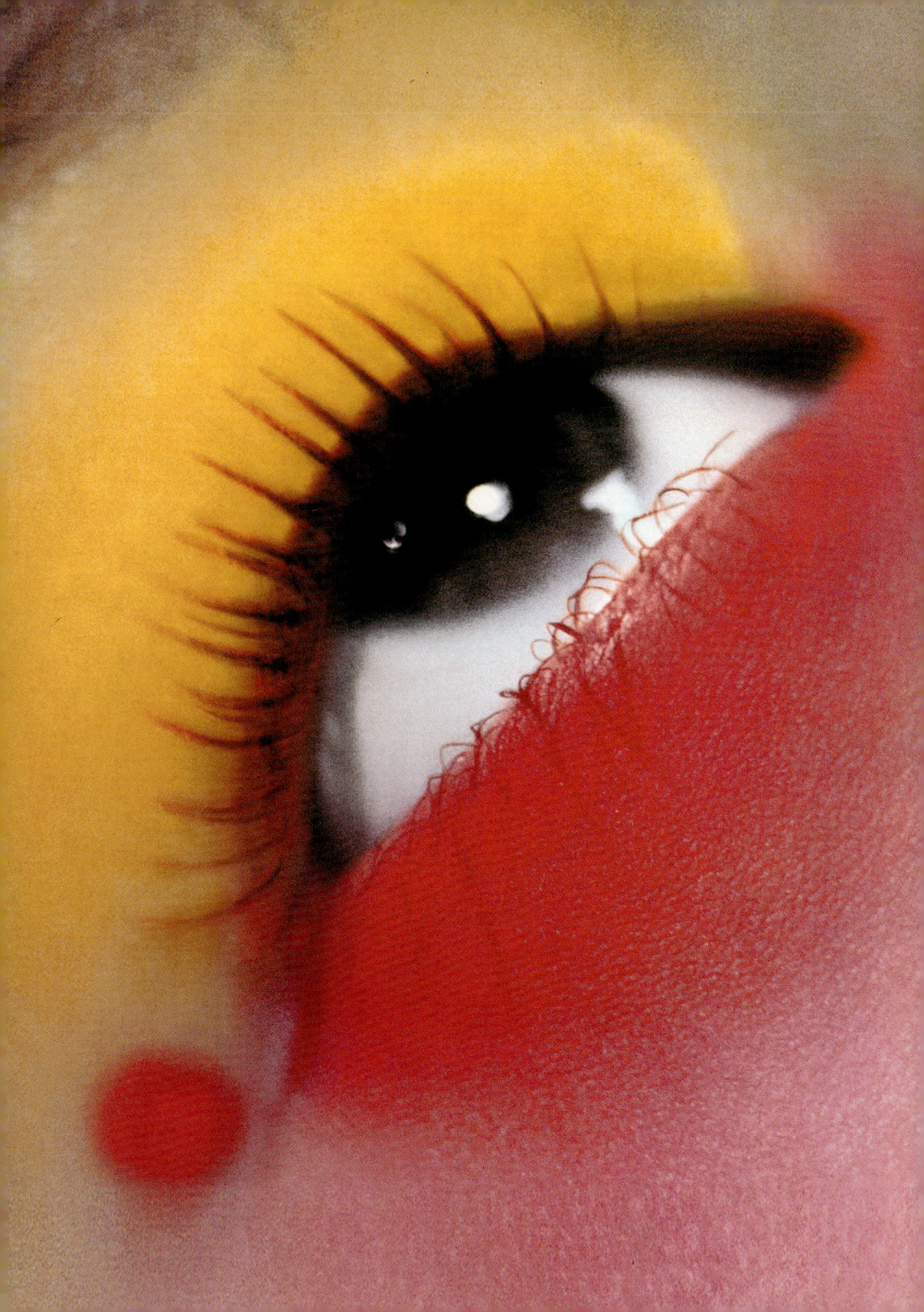

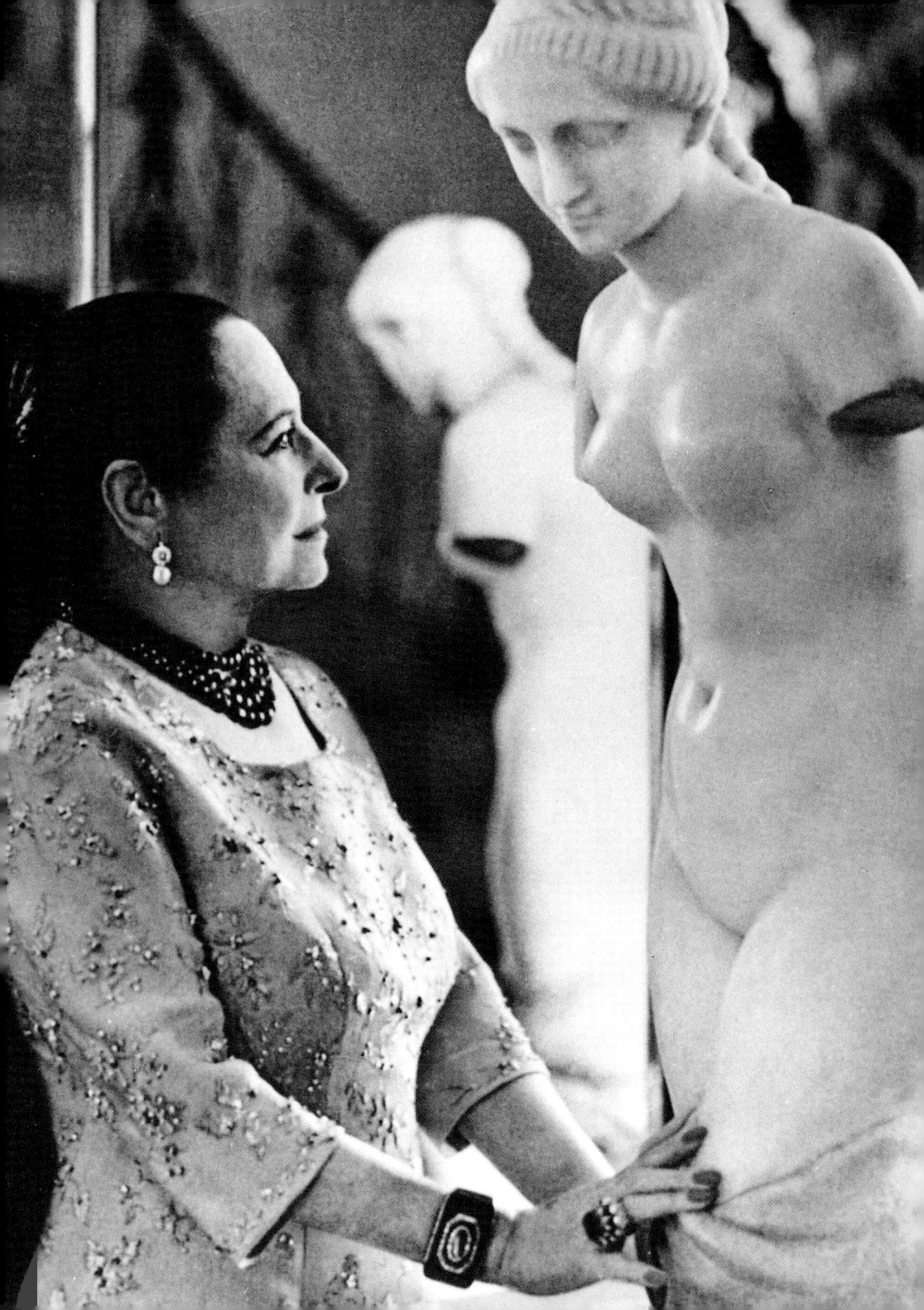

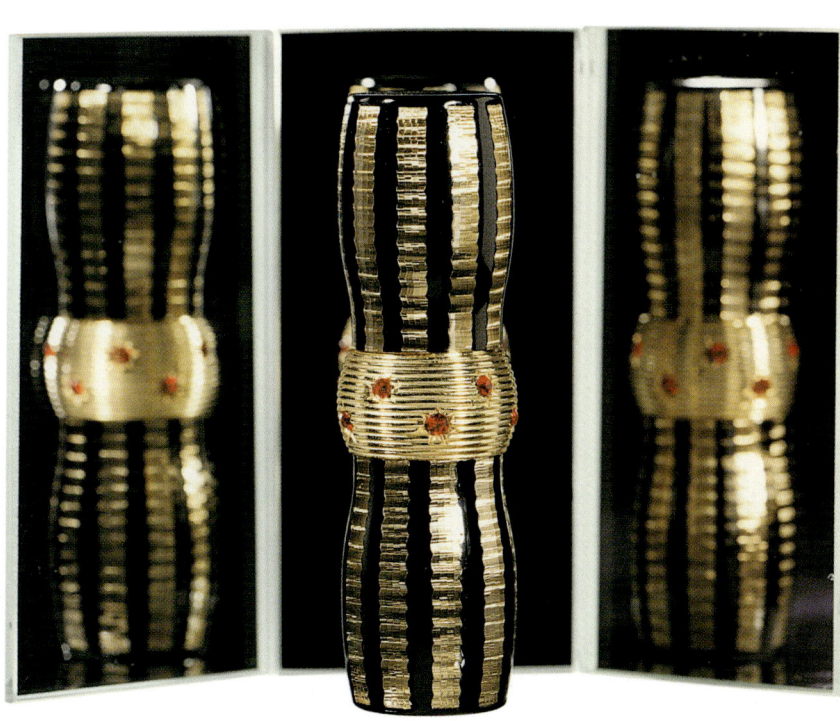

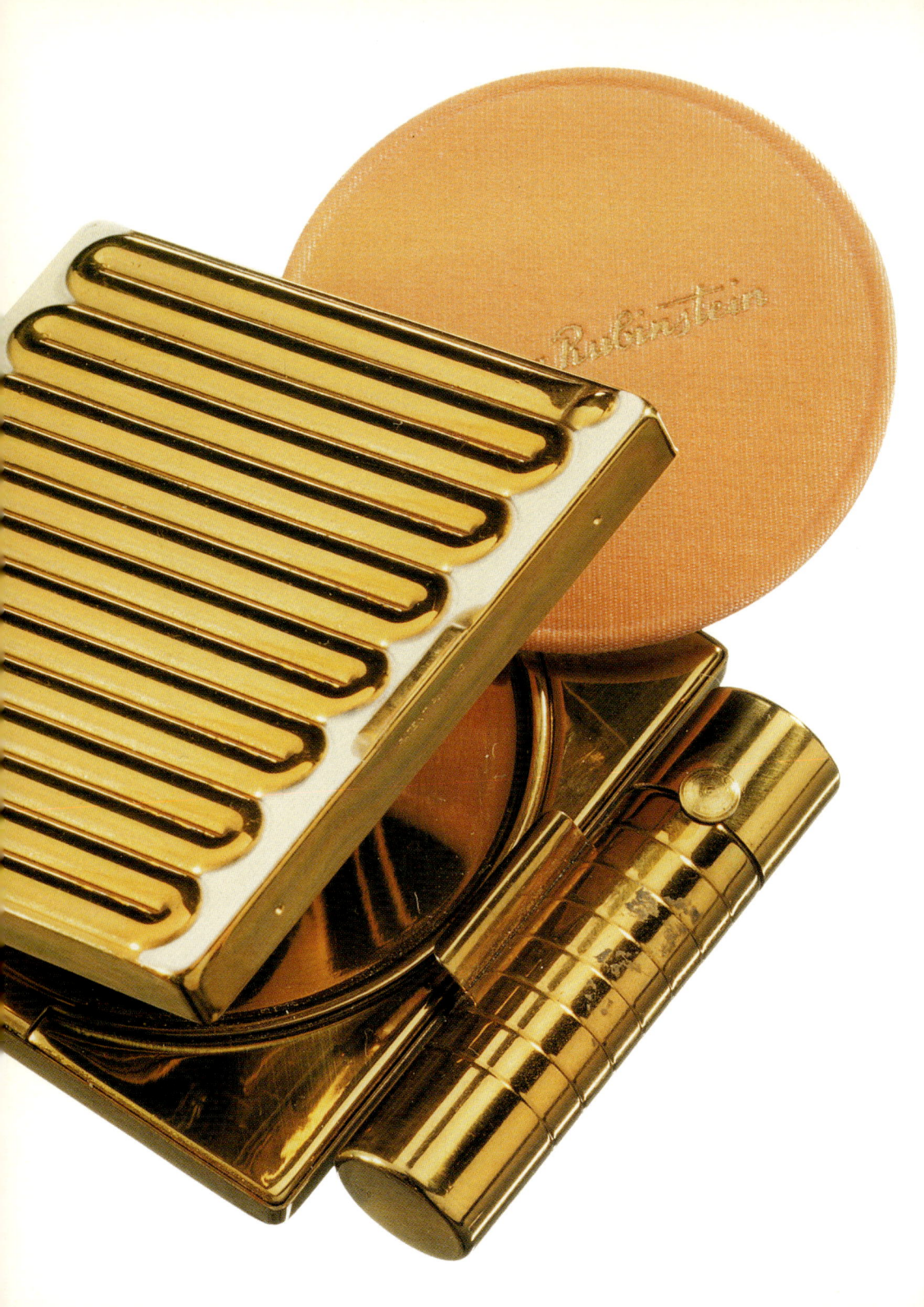

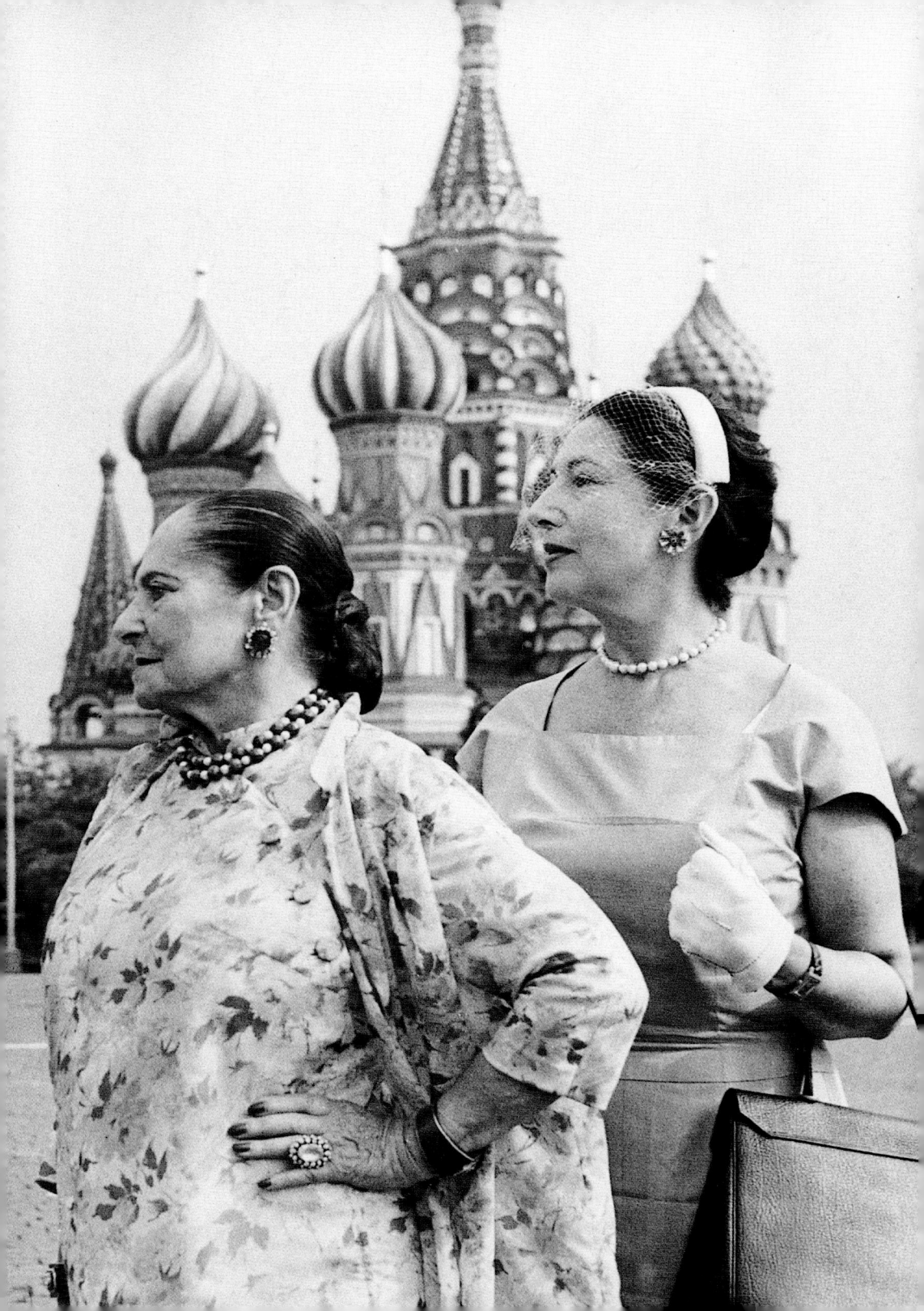

Helena Rubinstein
VALAZE
PASTEURIZED
CREAM
for Cleansing, Massage
and Nourishing
Valaze
Pasteurized
Facial Cream
VALAZE
FOR
BEAUTY

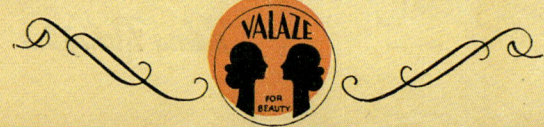

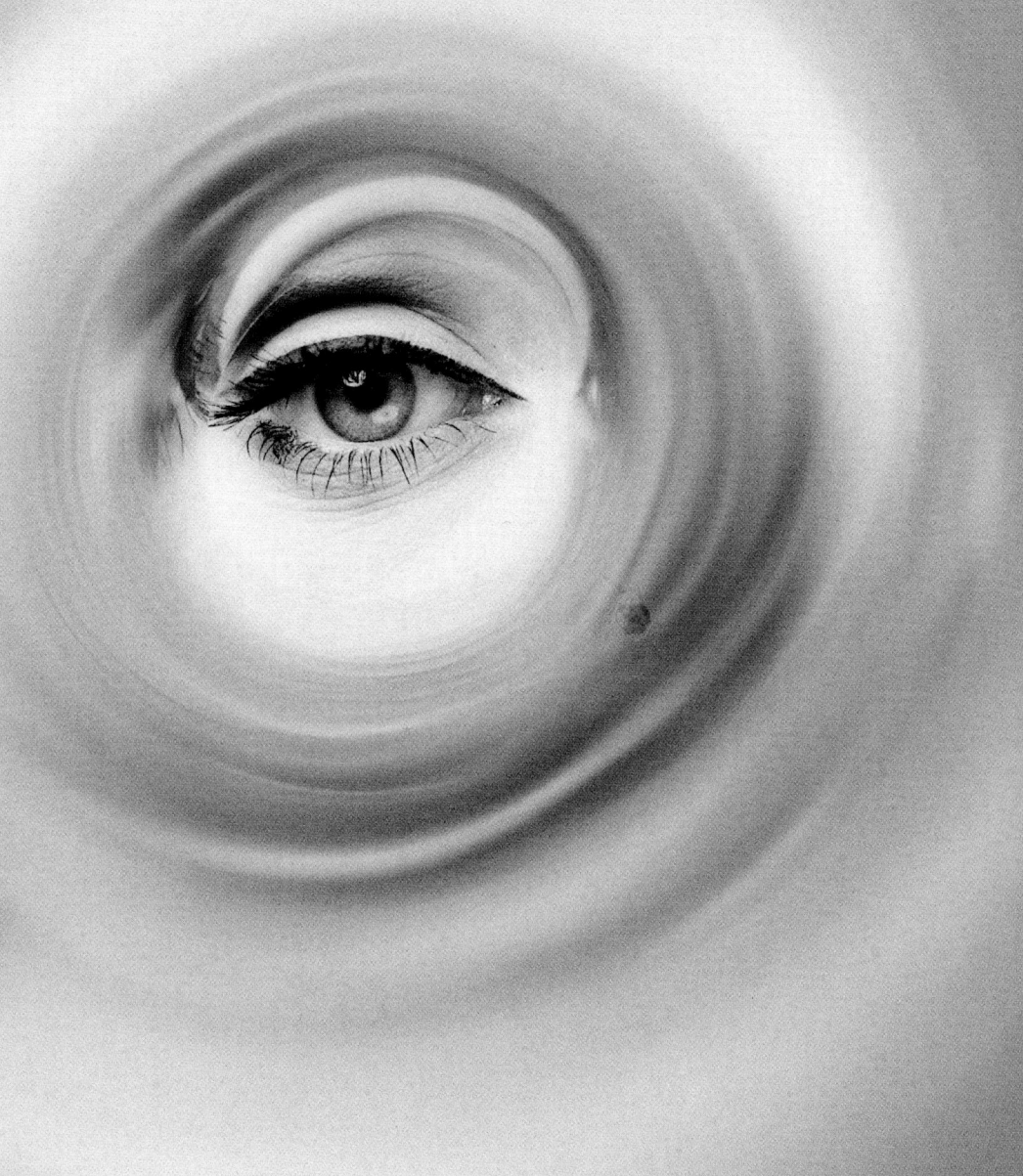

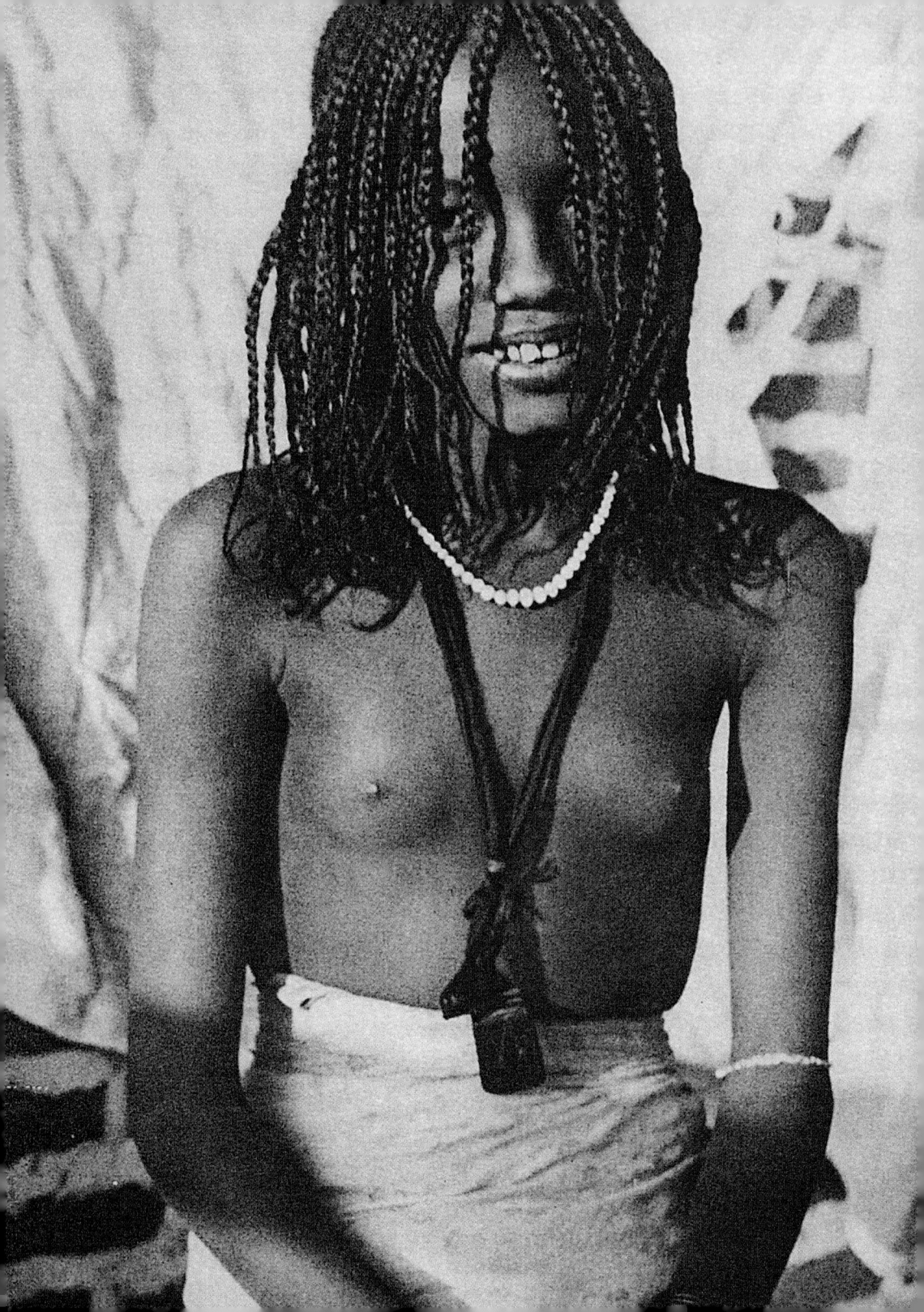

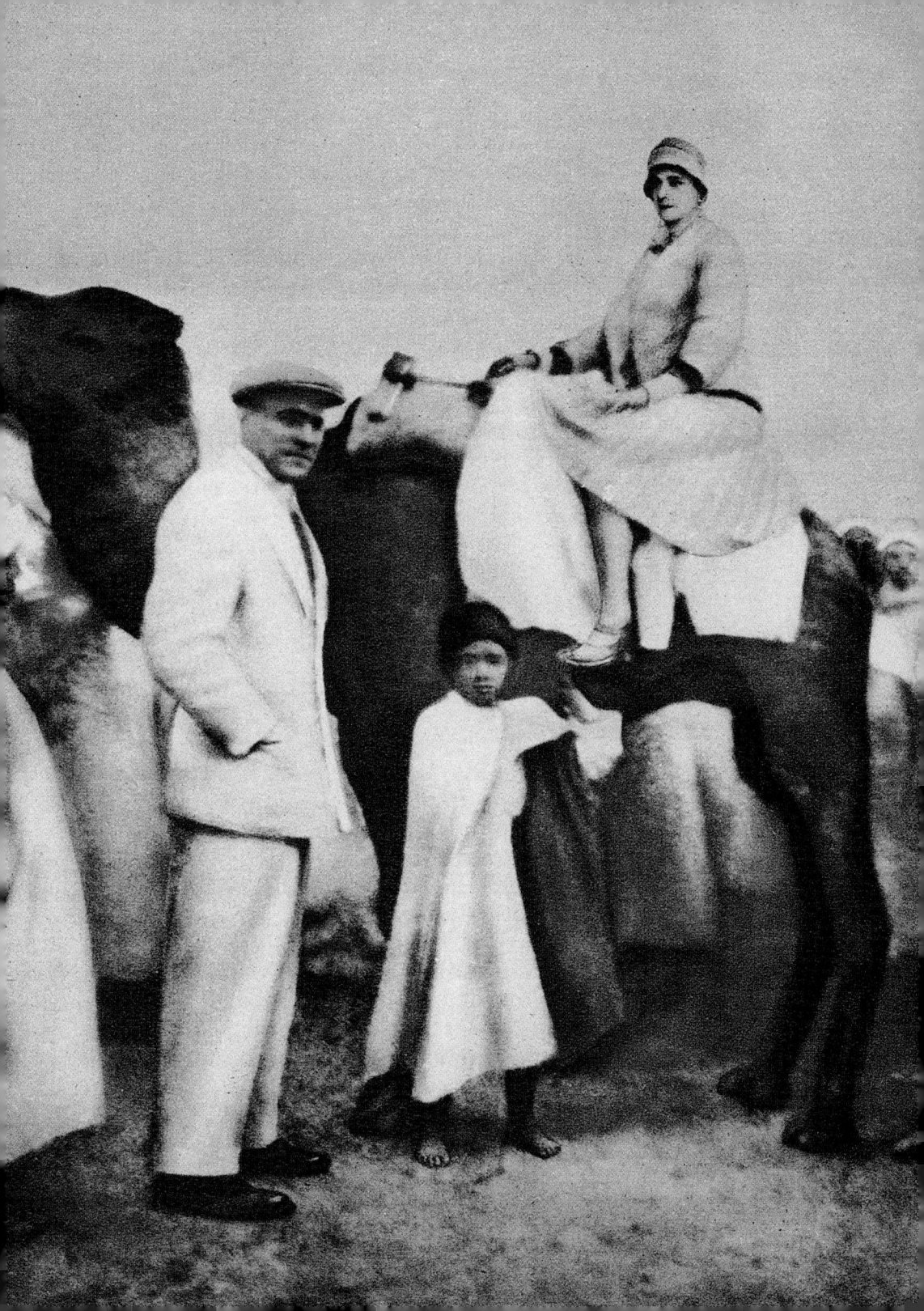

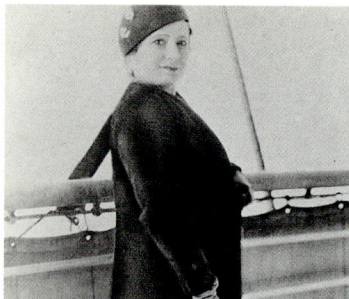
1930: Crossing the Atlantic in a Chanel suit.

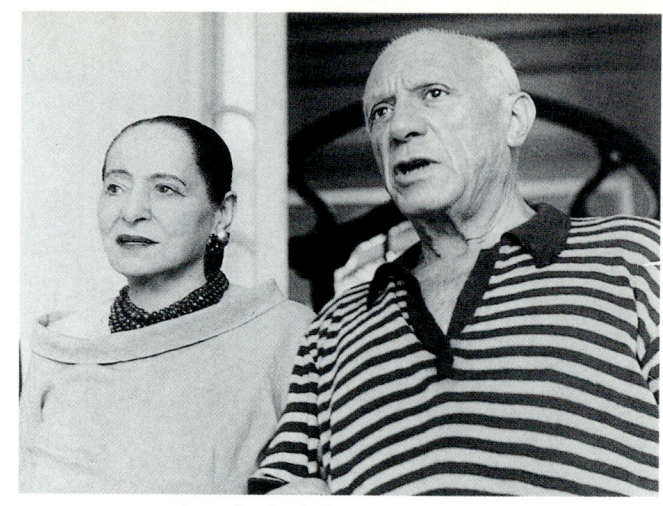
Picasso made 20 sketches for her portrait, but never finished it.

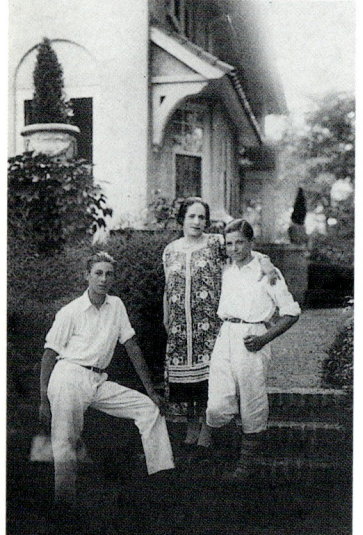
At Grasse, with her two sons, Ray and Horace.

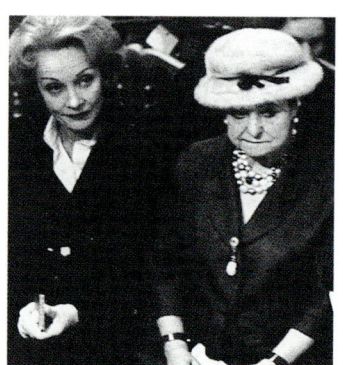
With Marlene Dietrich at a Christian Dior fashion show

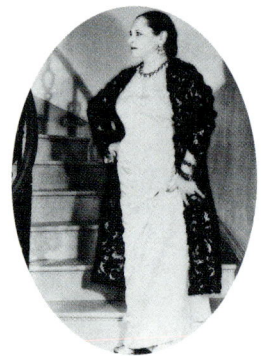
An aquiline profile and a thoughtful expression, 1927.

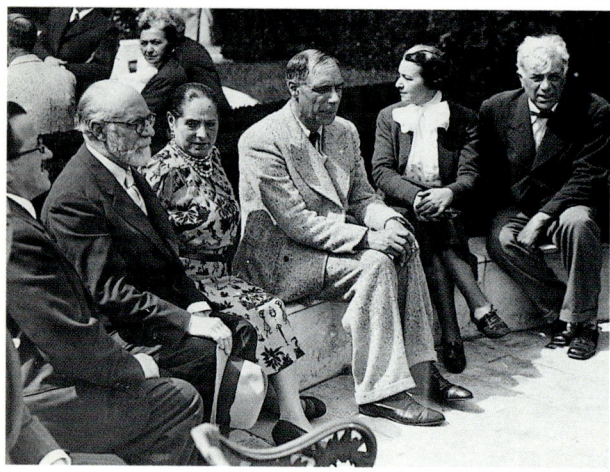
The Rubinstein clan.

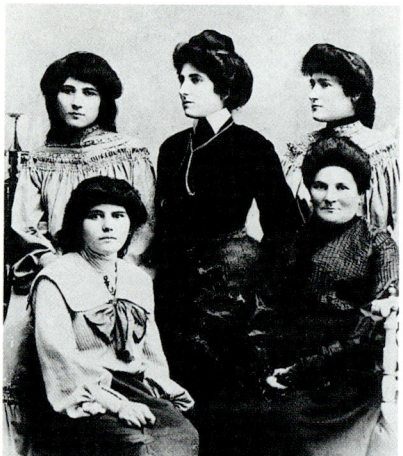
With her mother and sisters.

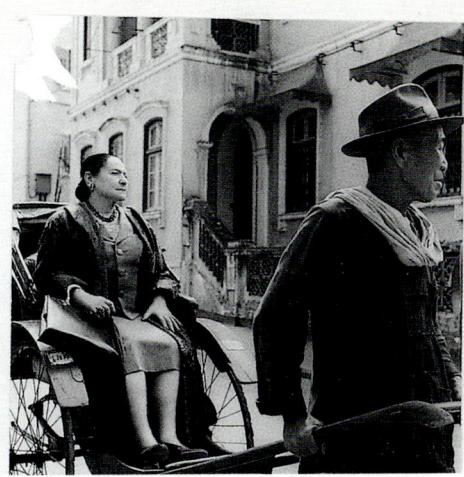
A trip to the far East, Hong Kong, 1957.

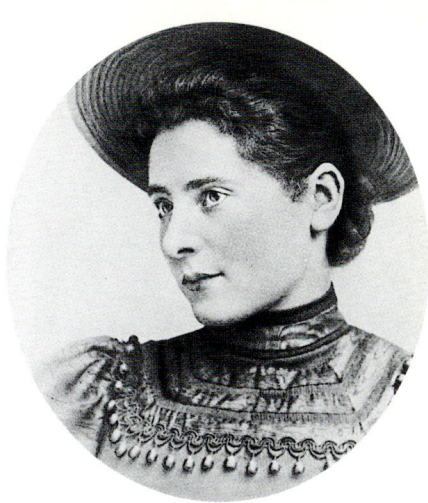
Helena as a young girl in Cracow.

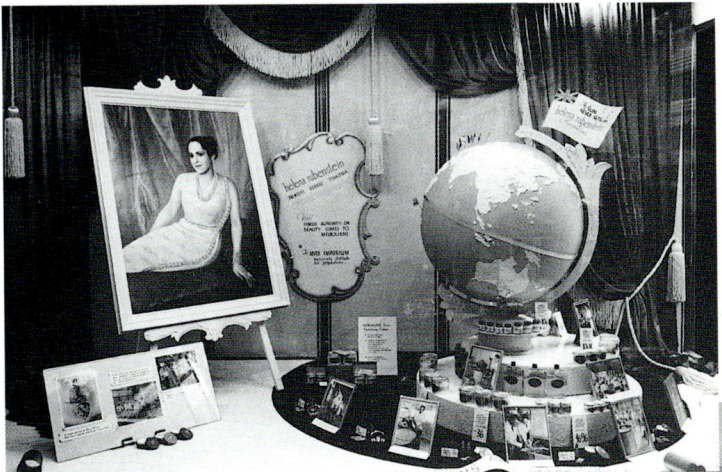
Her portrait in the window of a New-York department store.

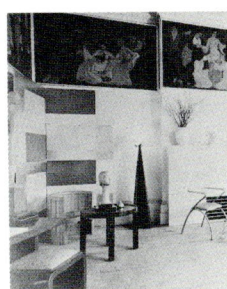
Esthete philantropist, friend of Matisse, Braque, Léger...

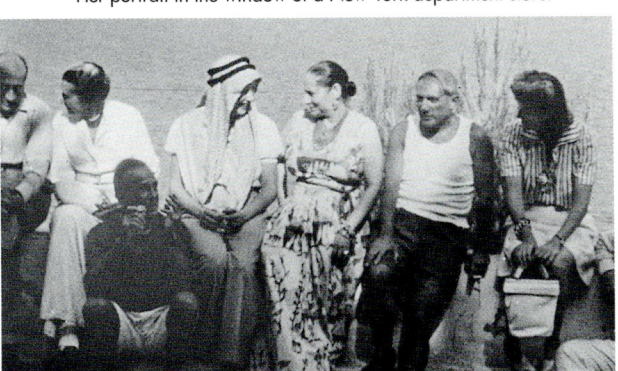
Pre-World War II, including Picasso, in Antibes.

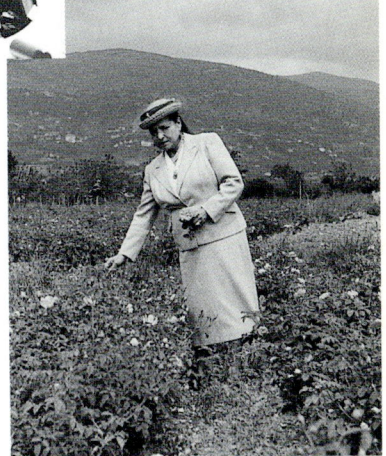
At Grasse, among her fields of jasmine

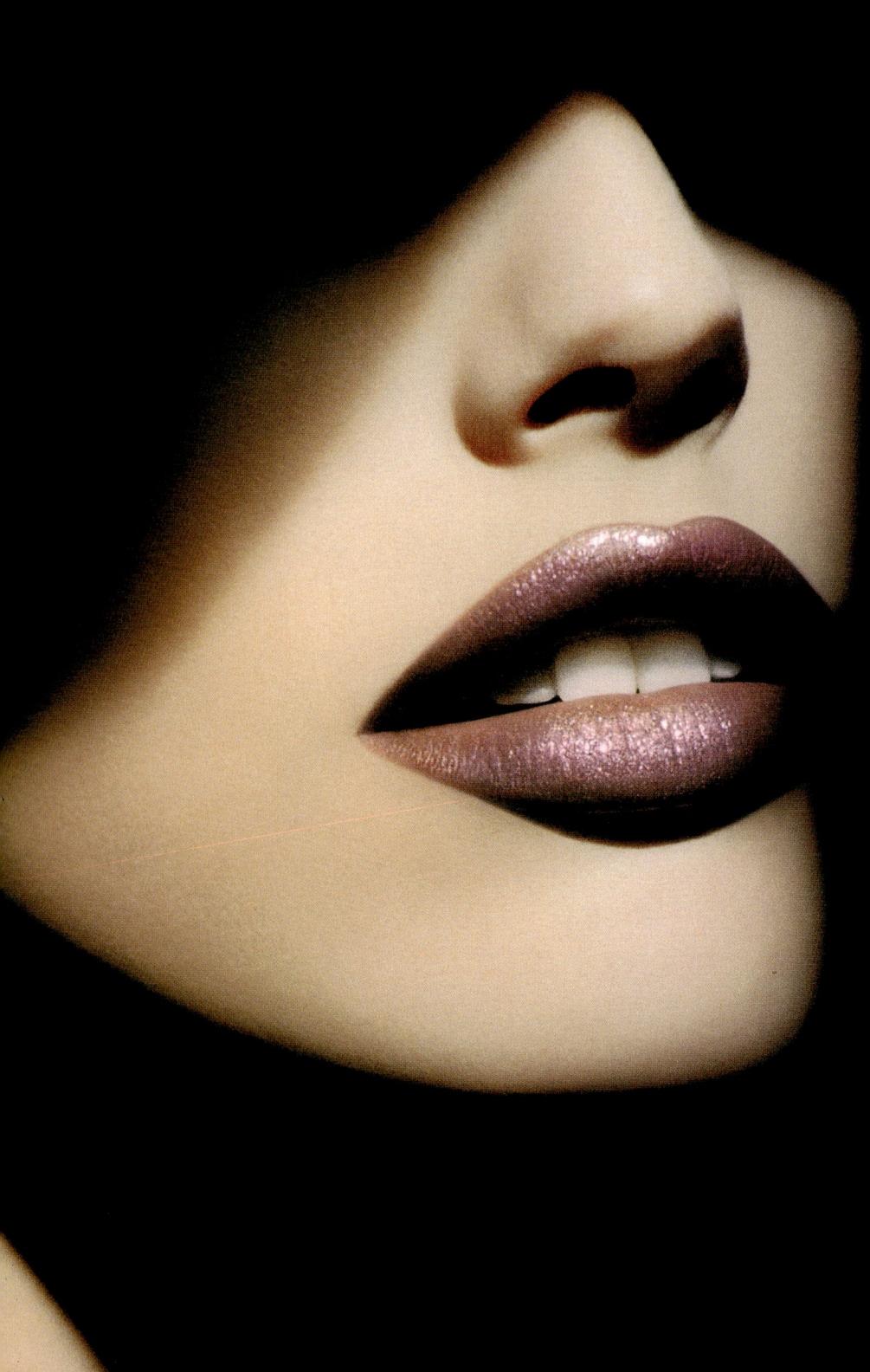

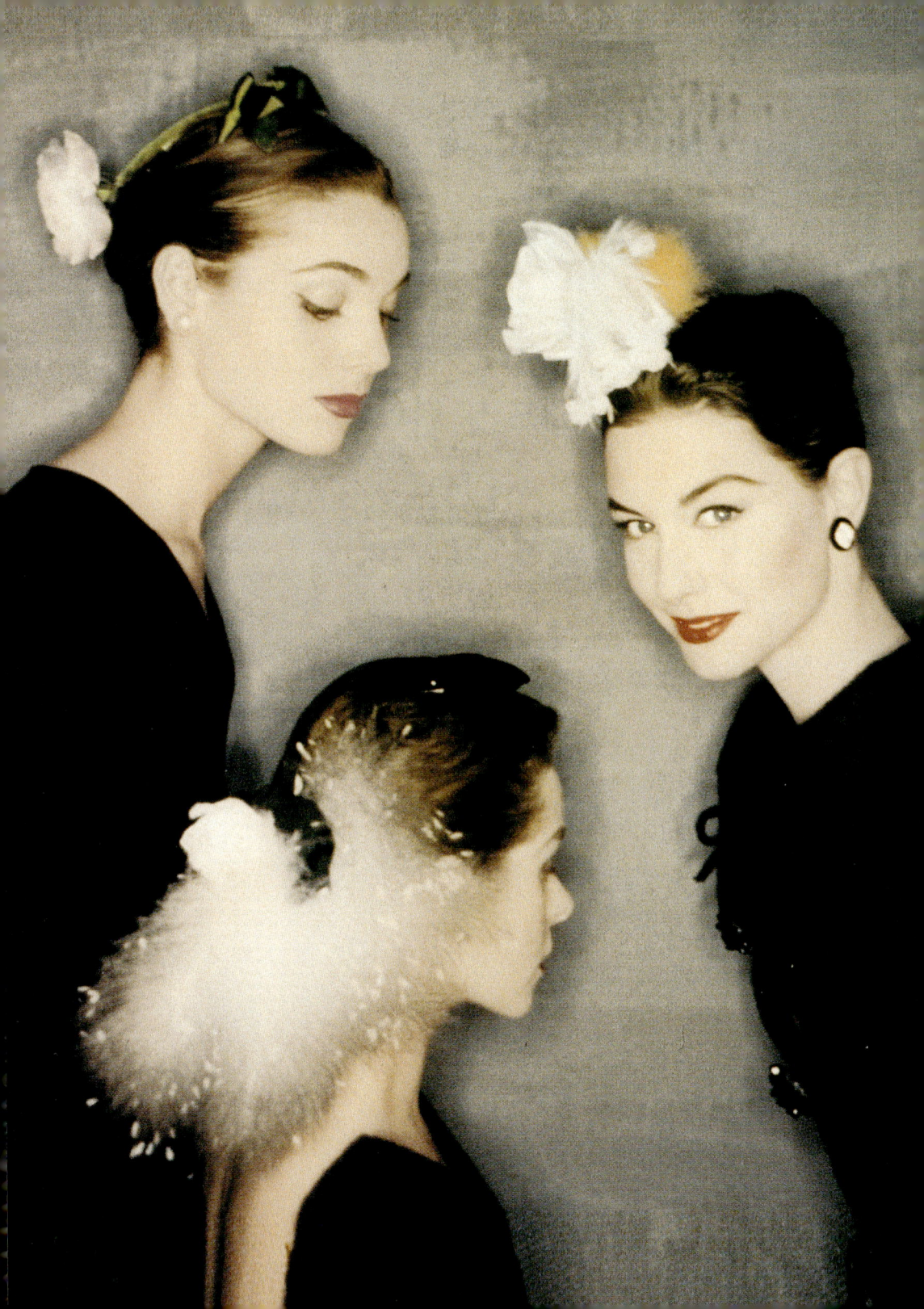

Helena Ru...

APPLE BLOSSOM

helena

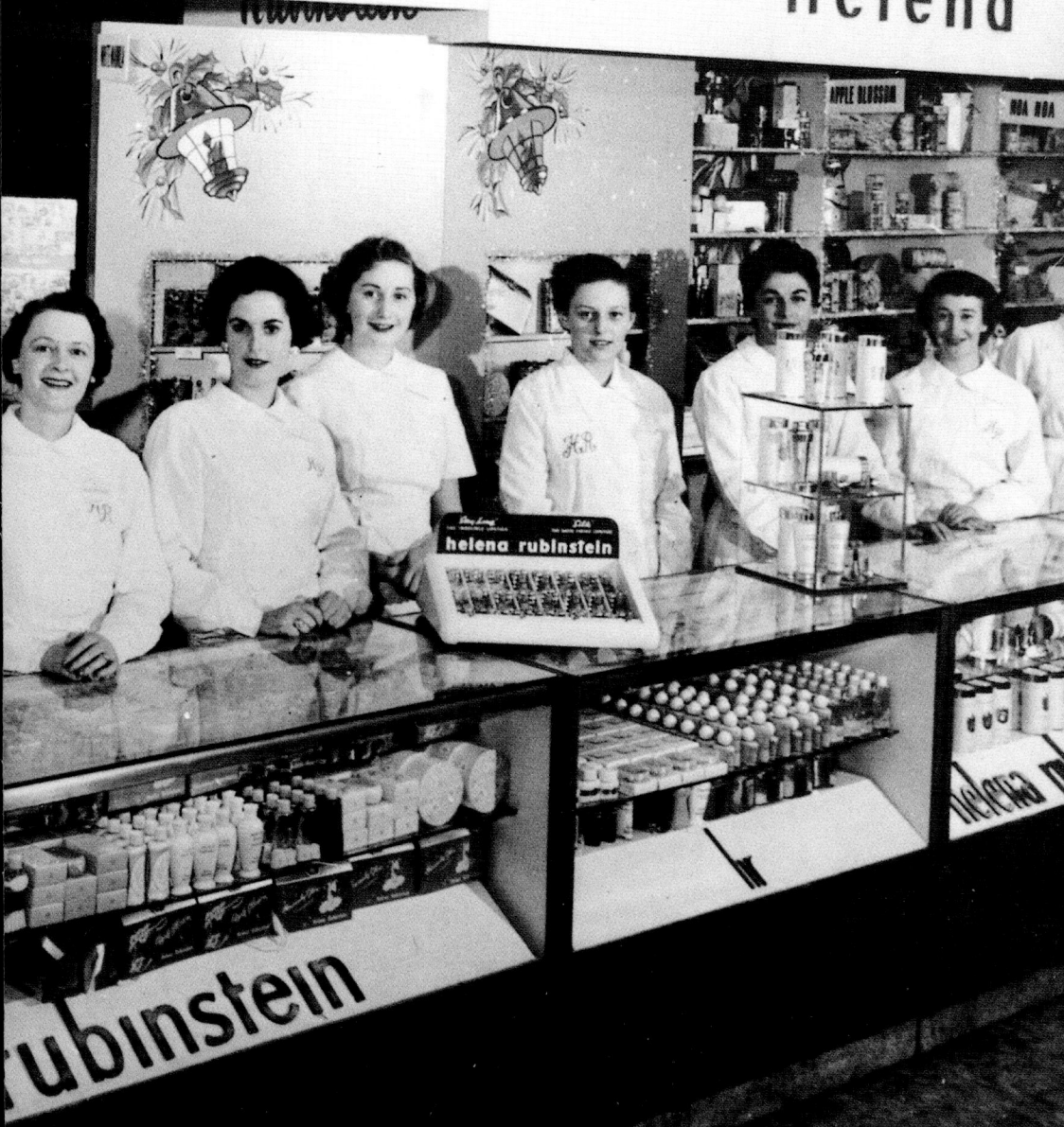

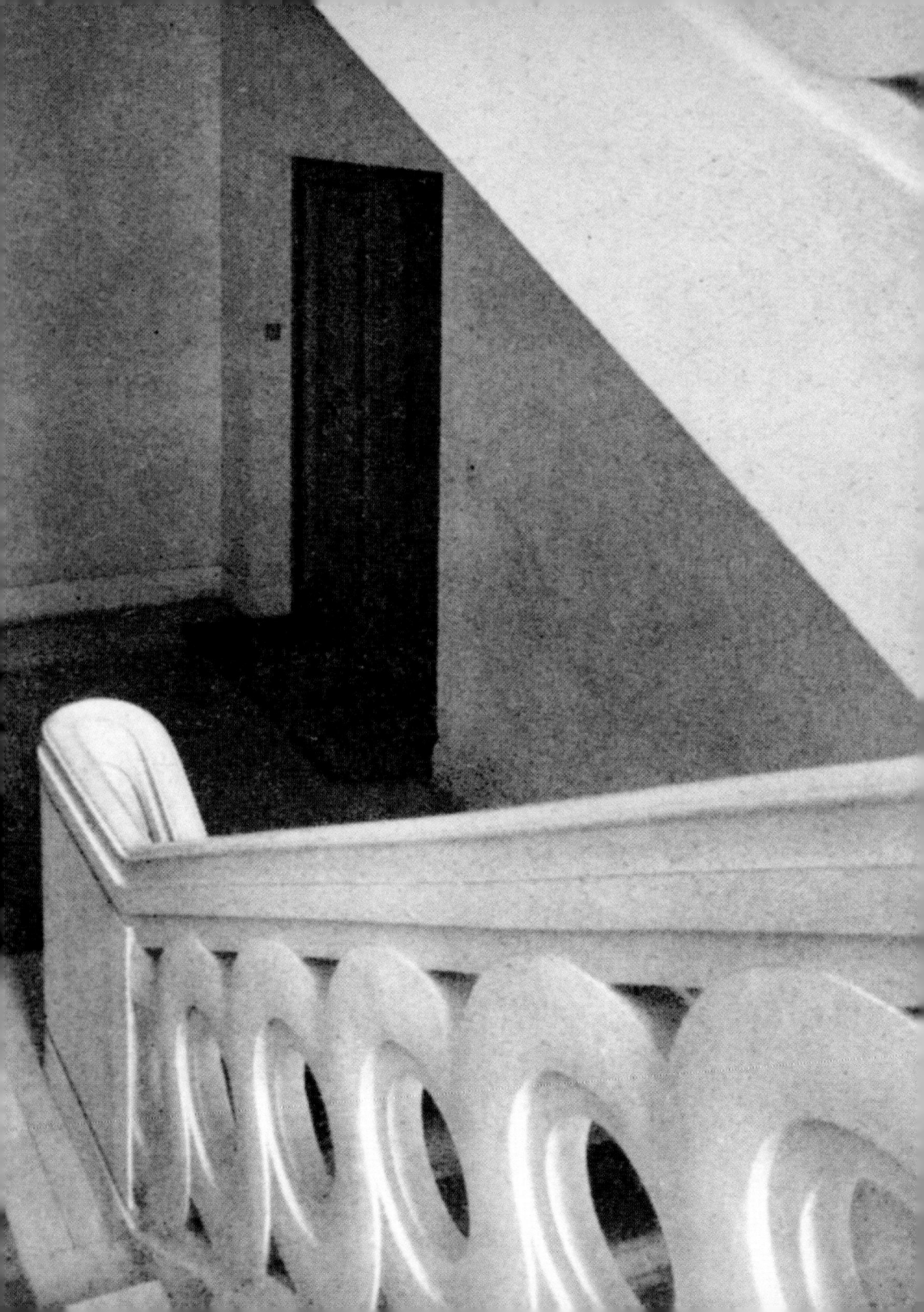

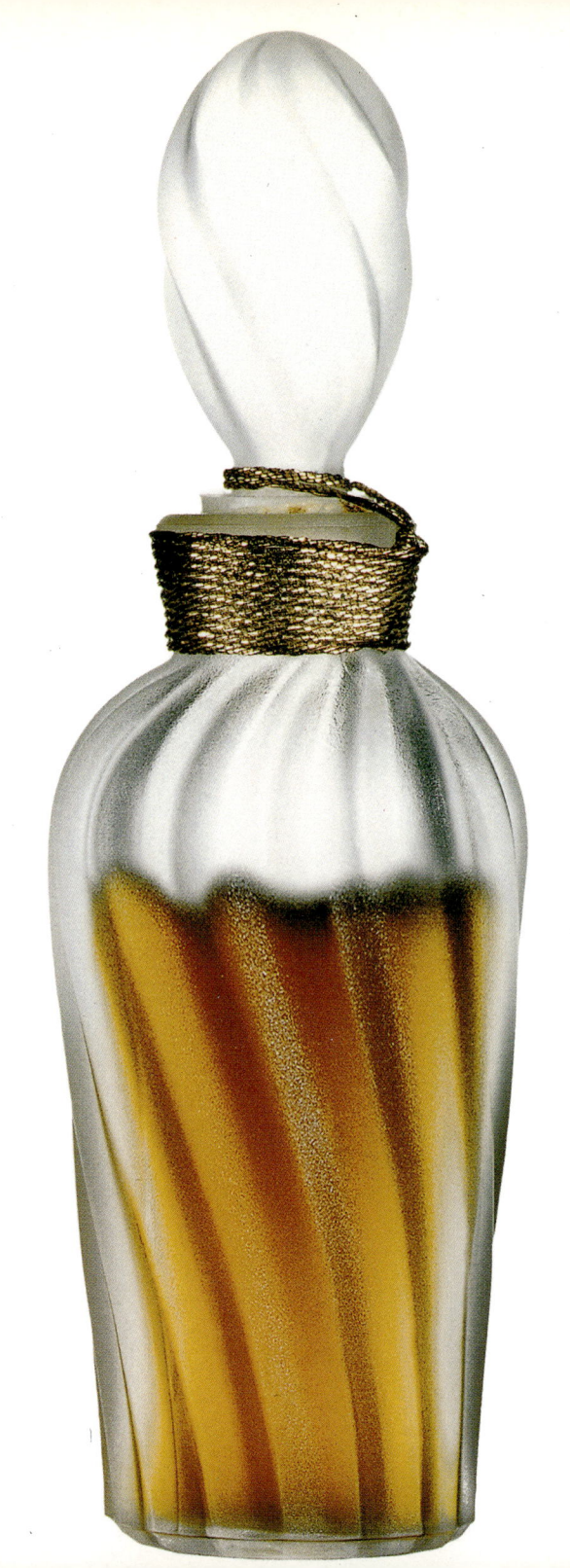

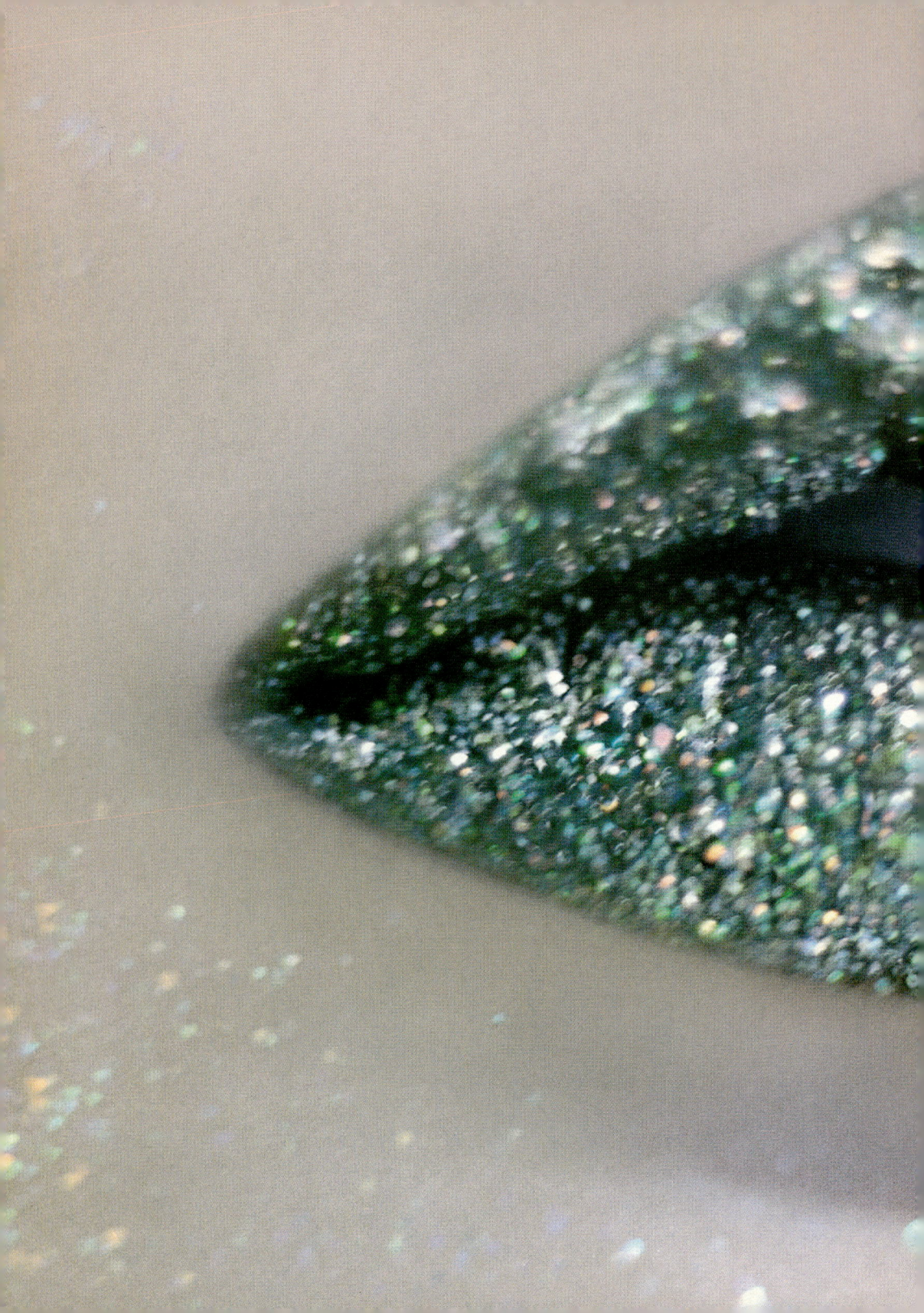

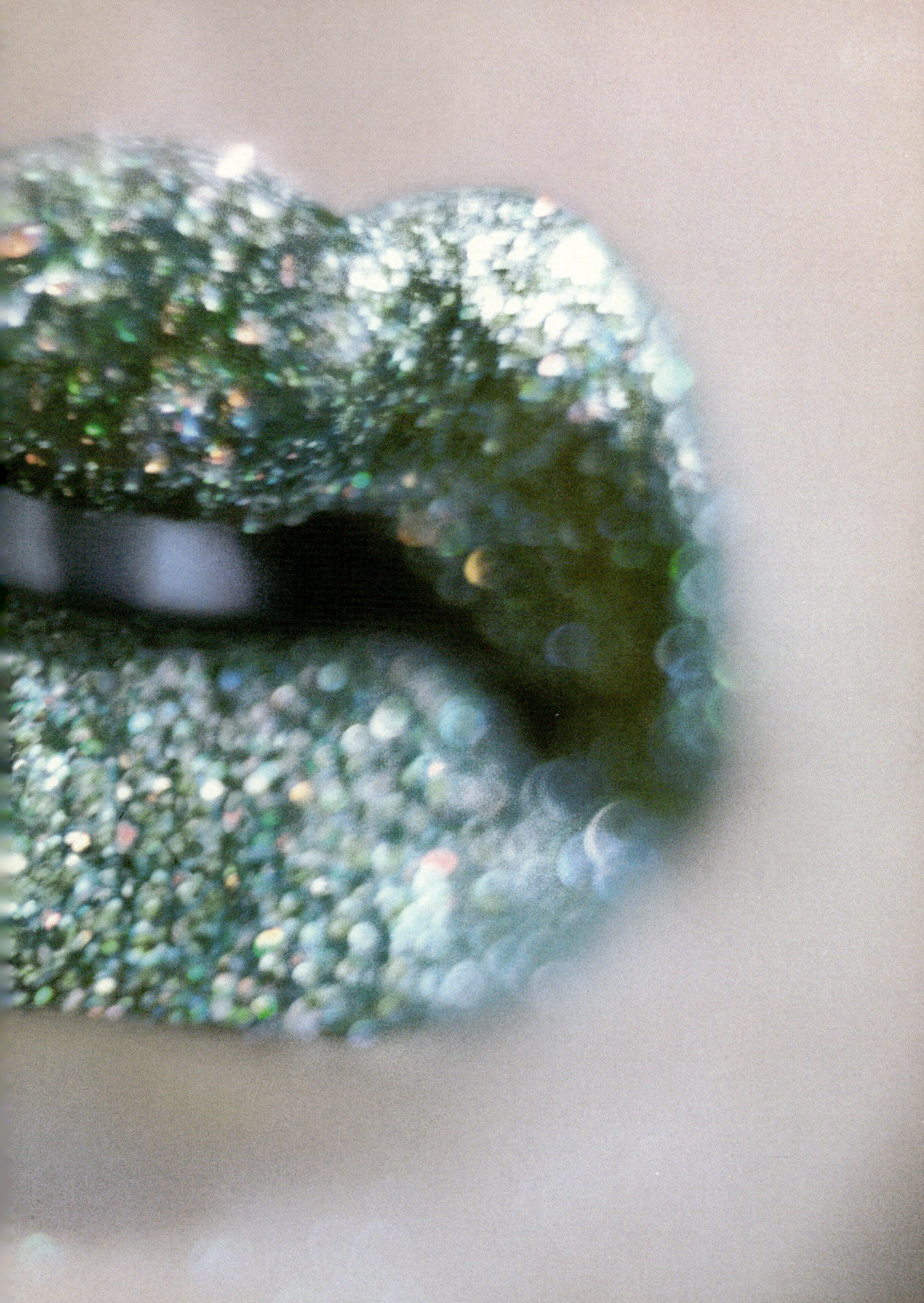

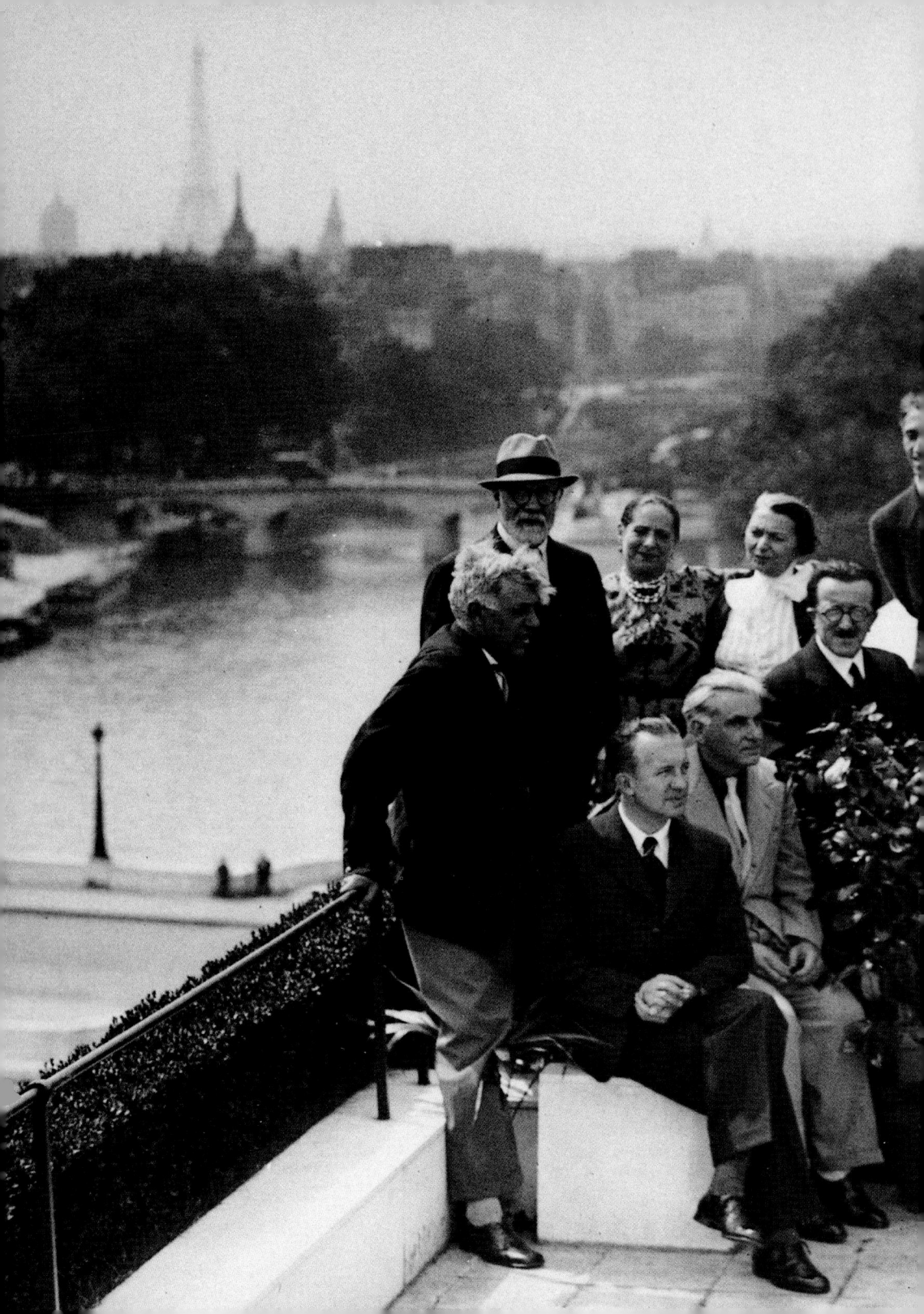

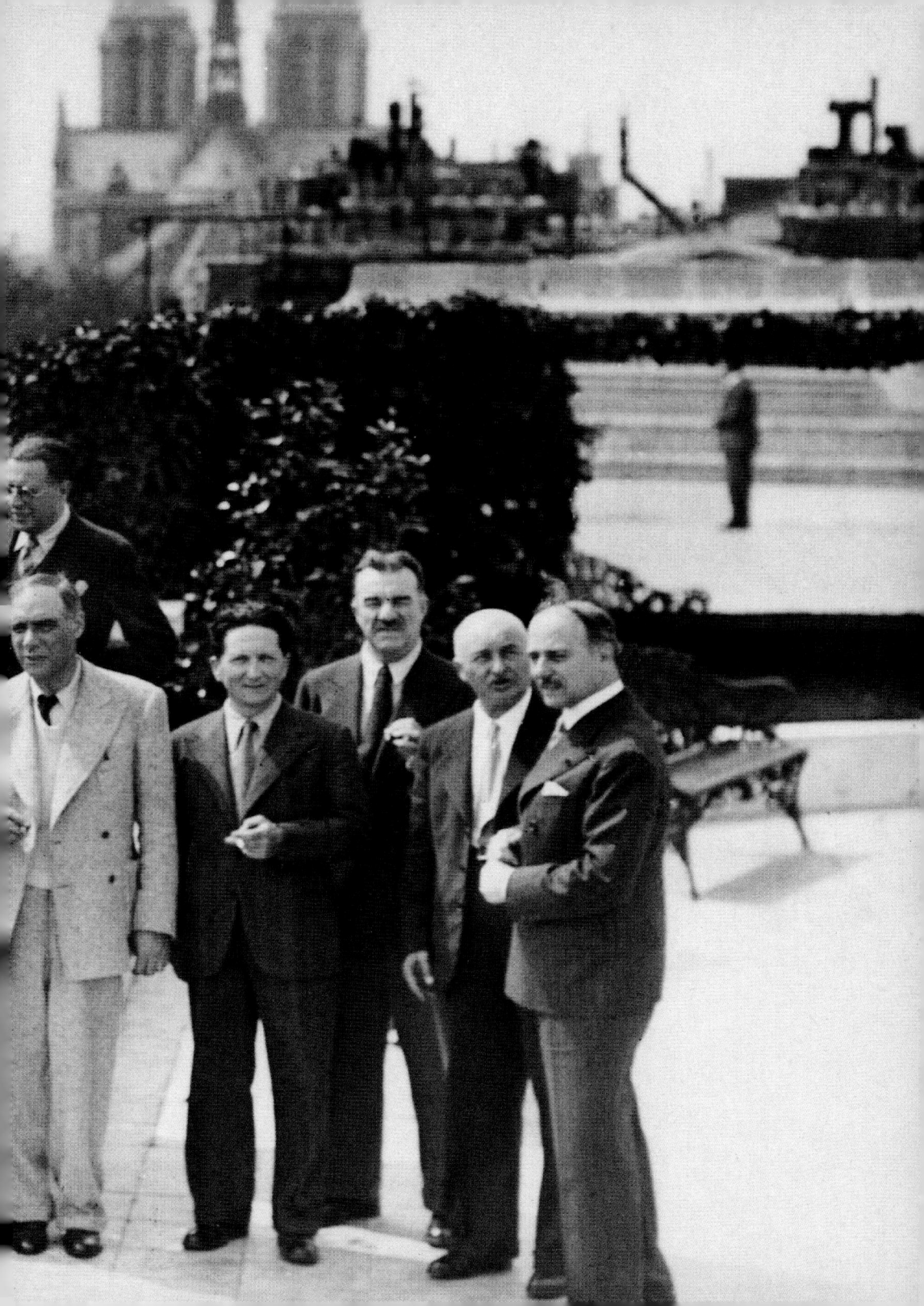

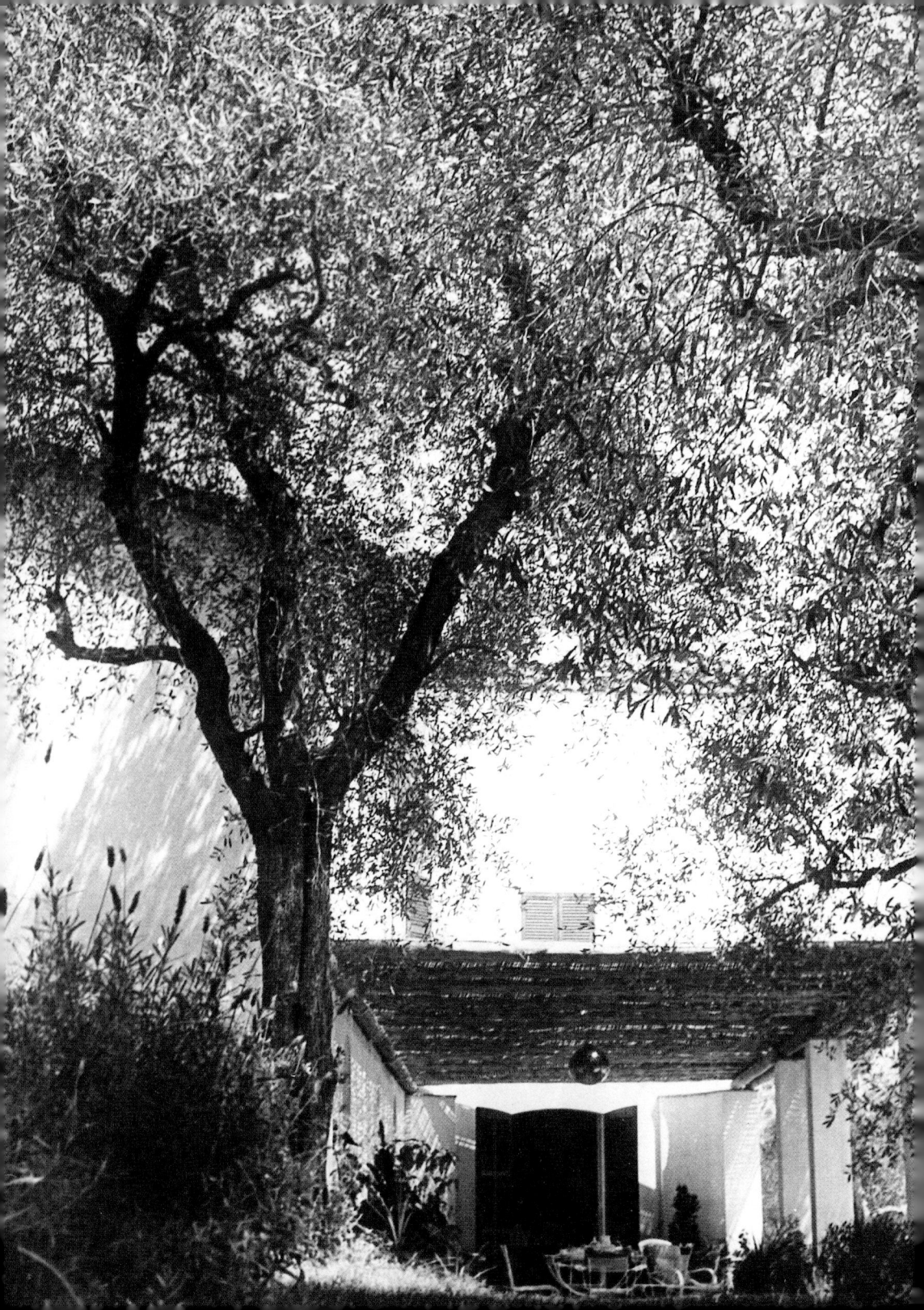

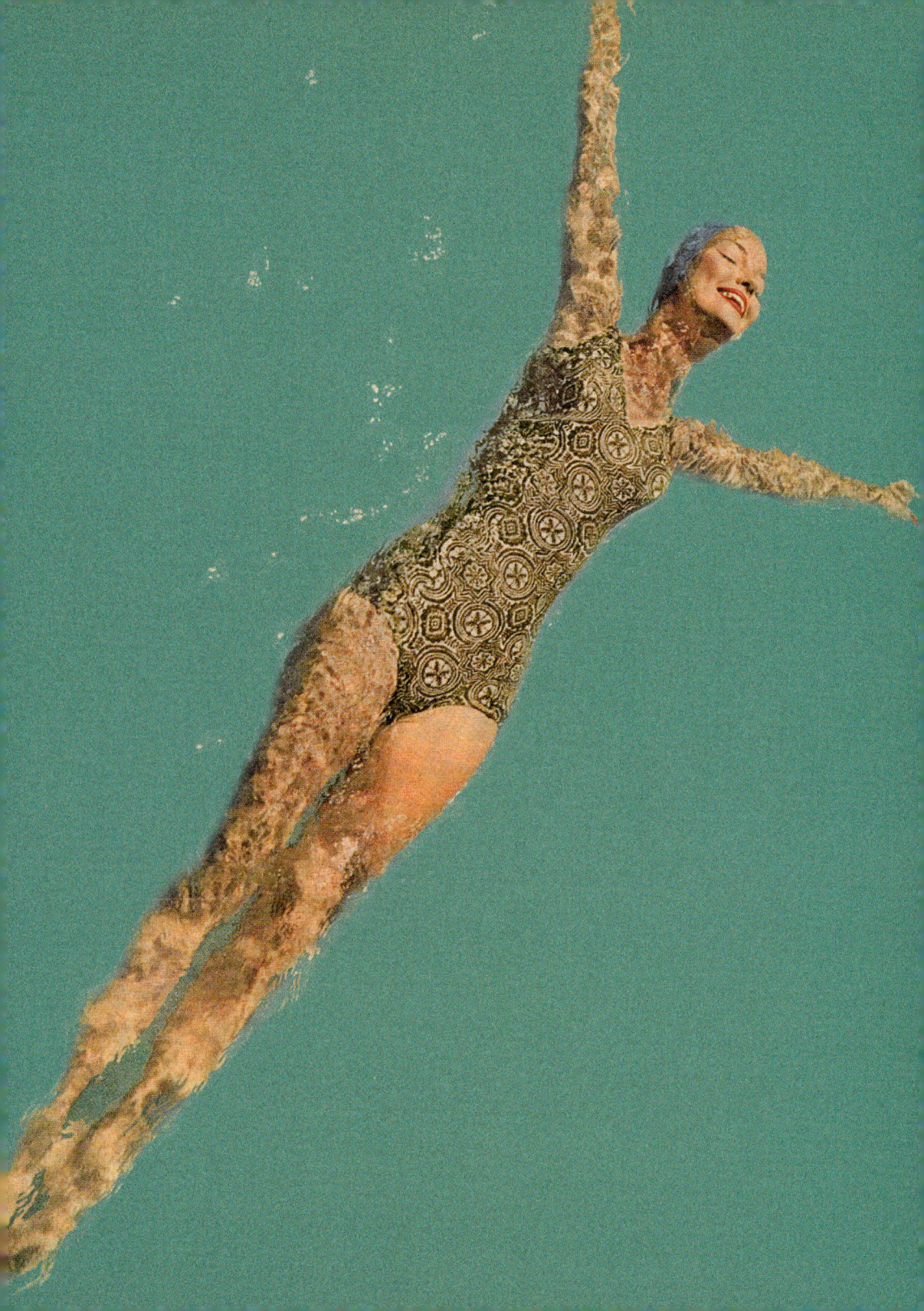

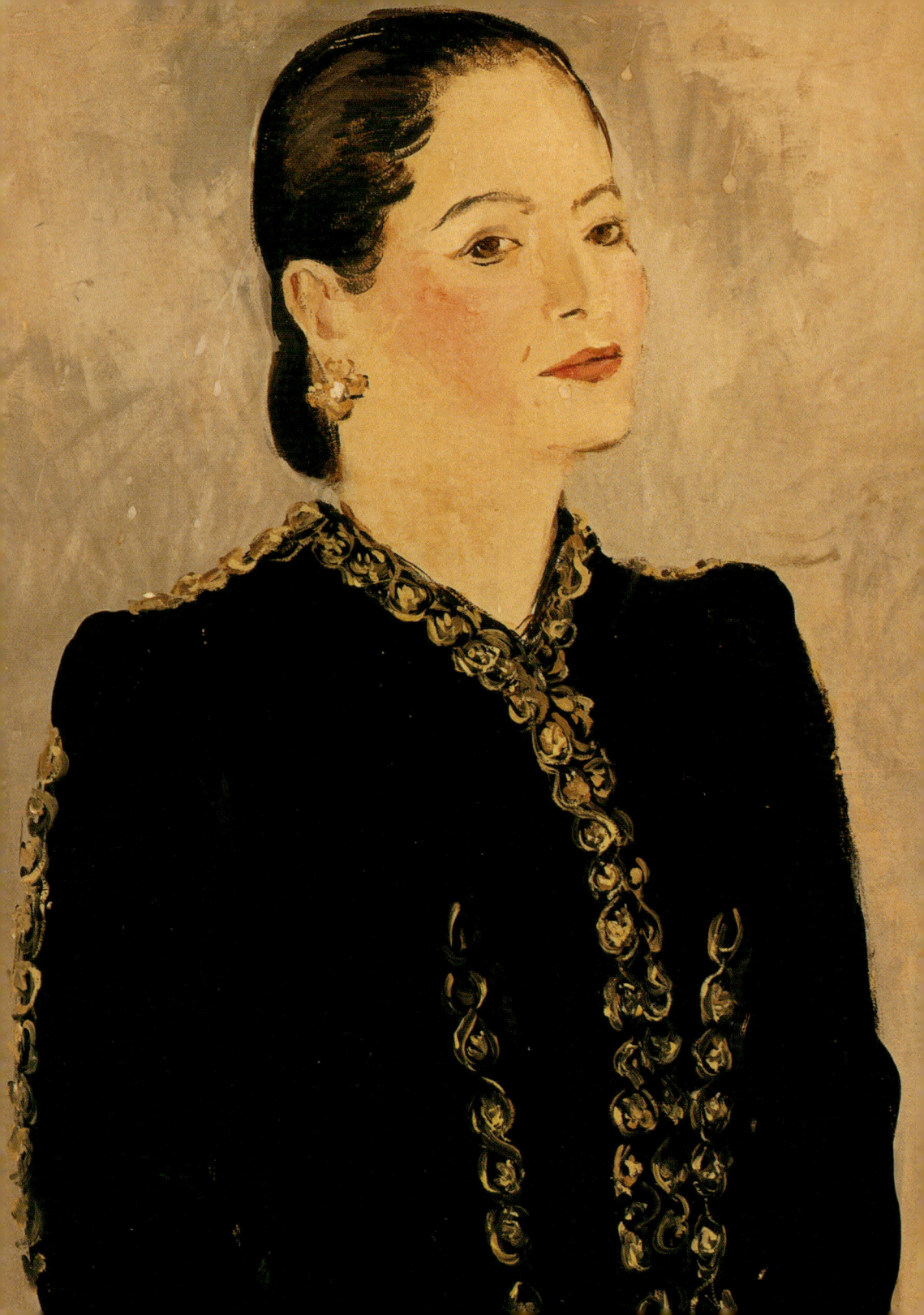

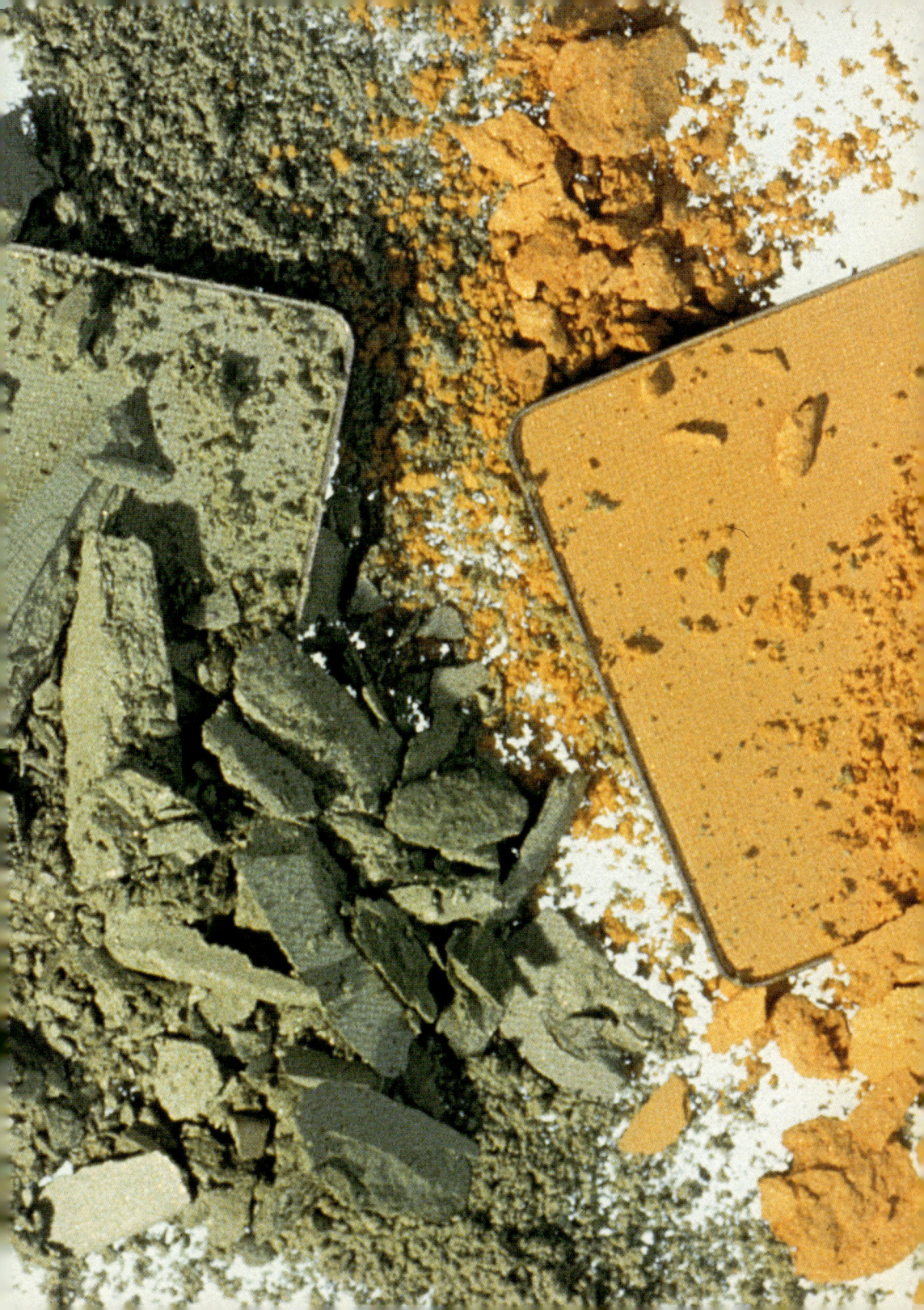

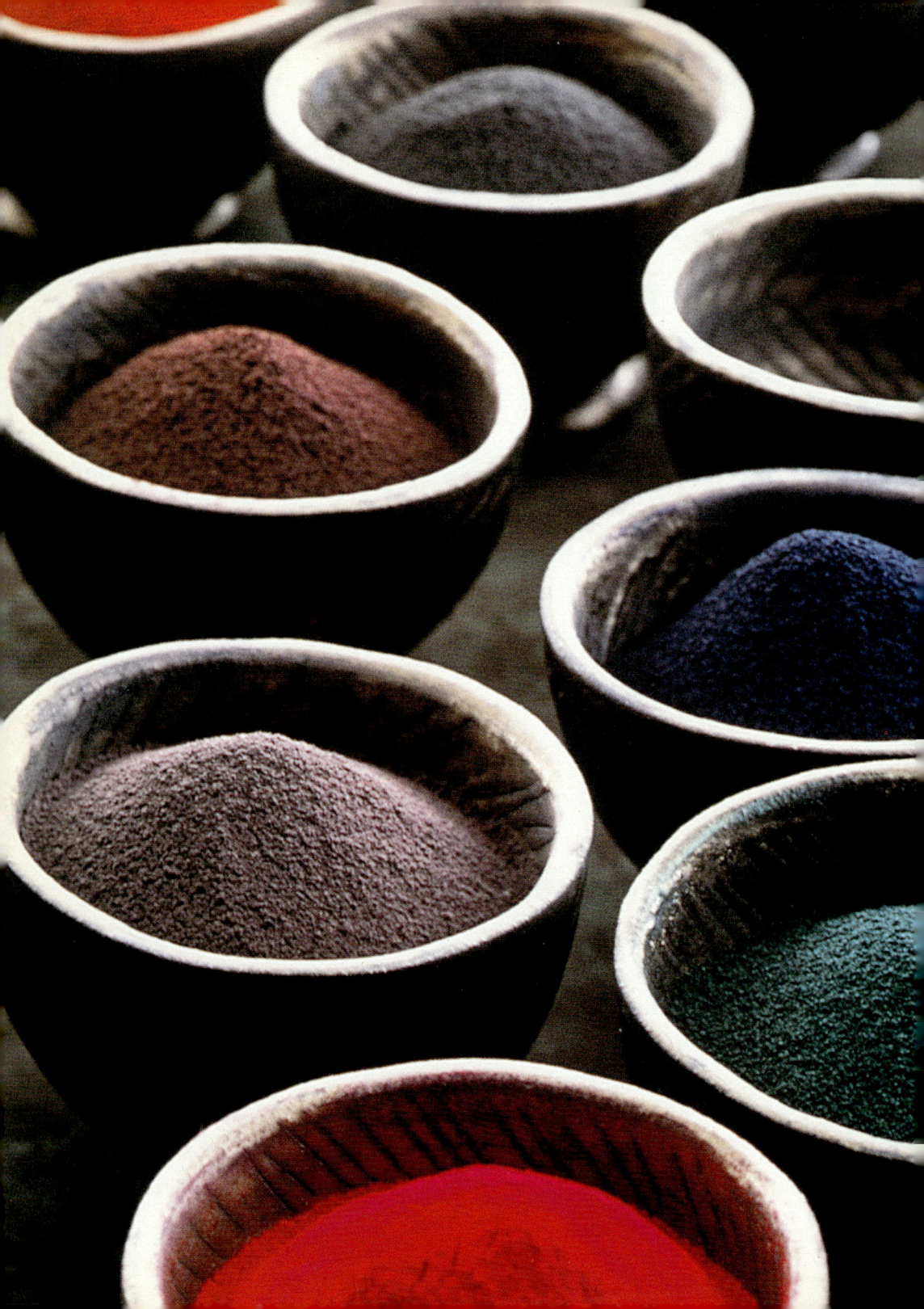

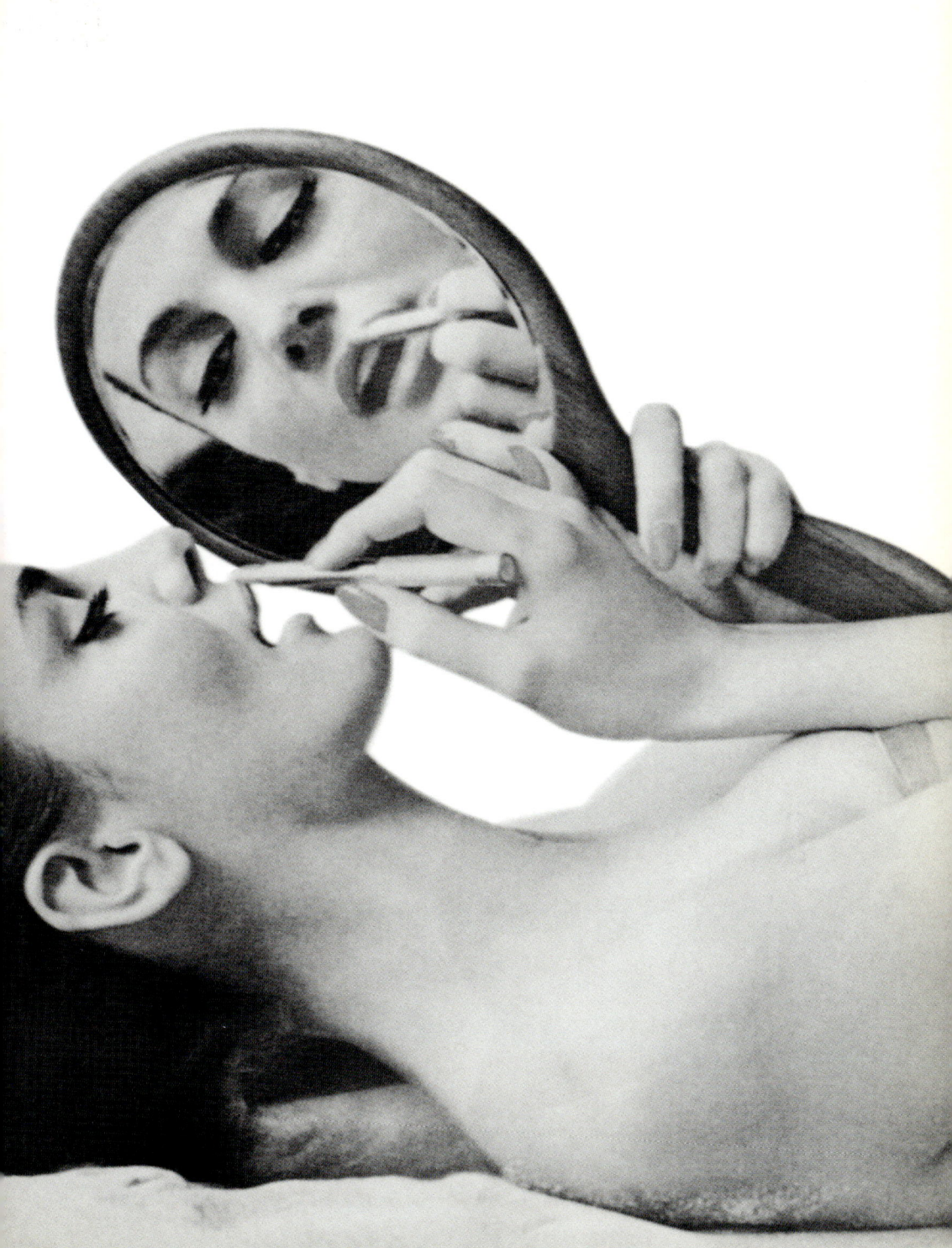

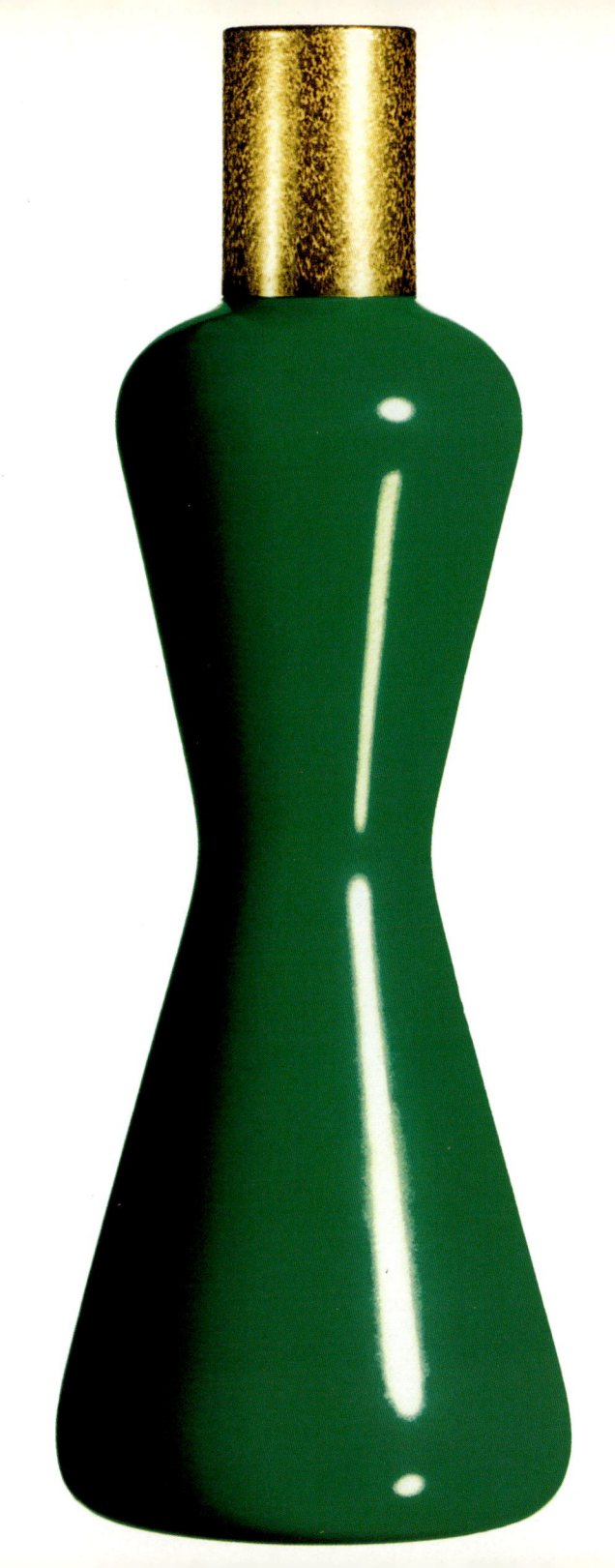

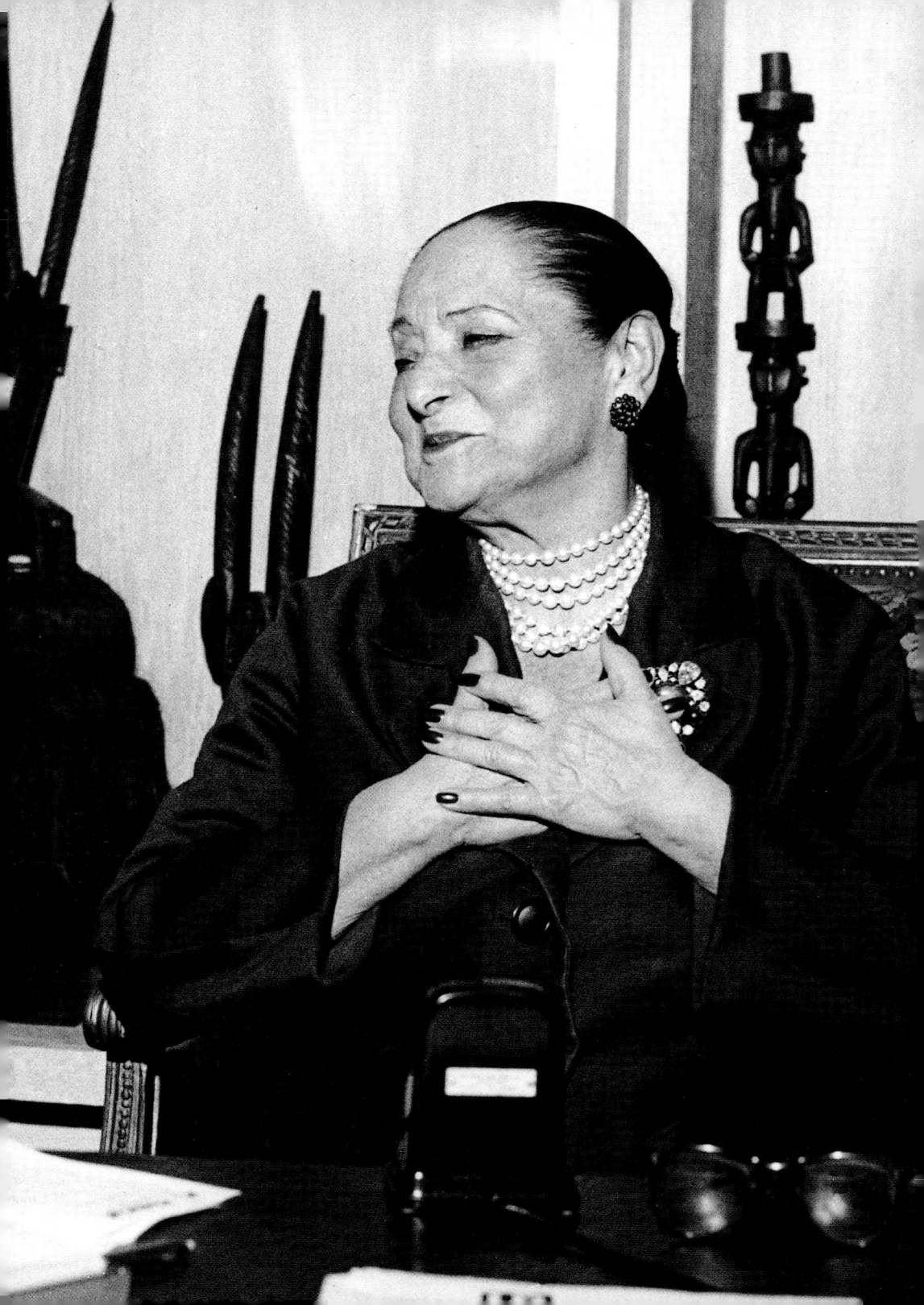

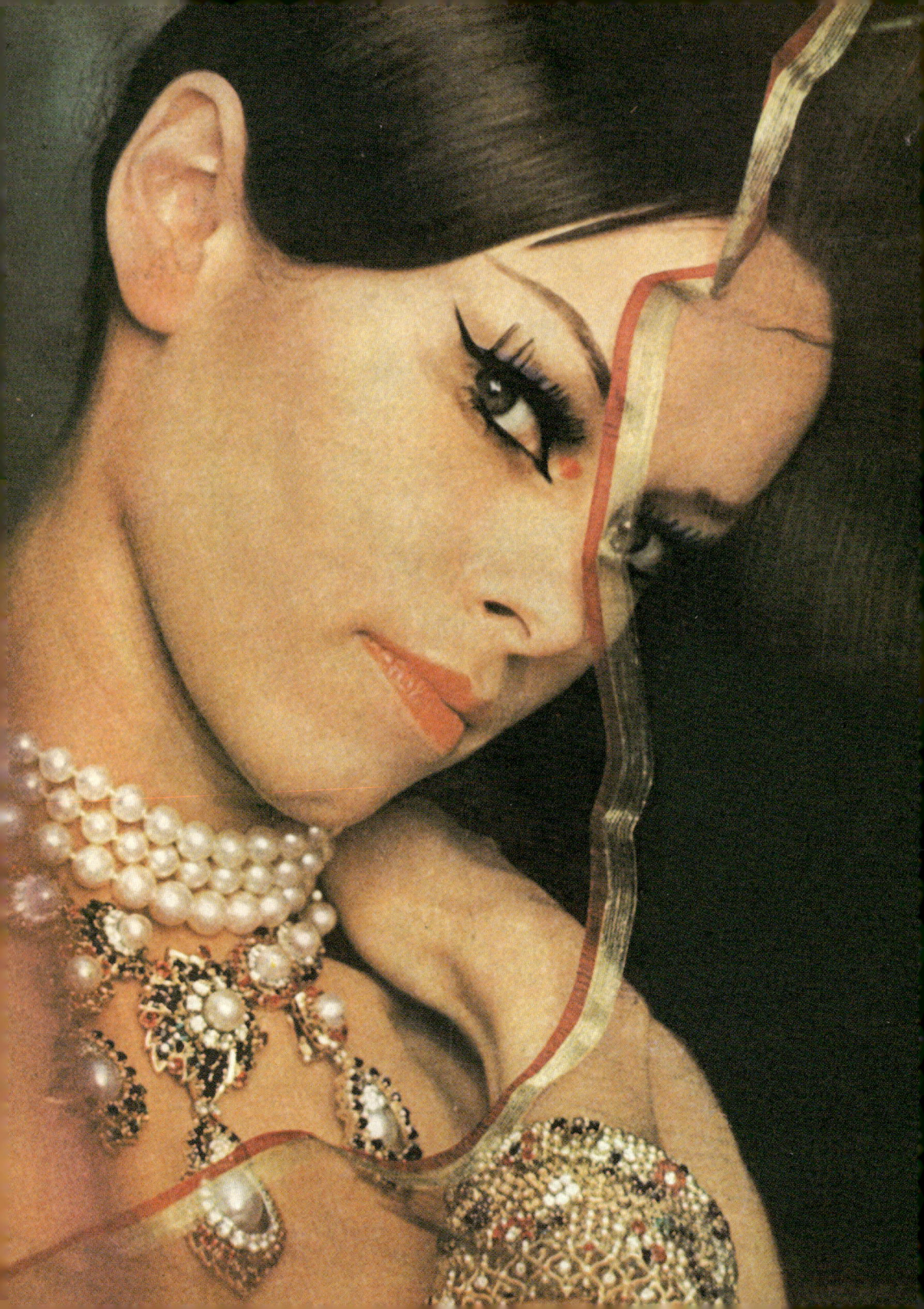

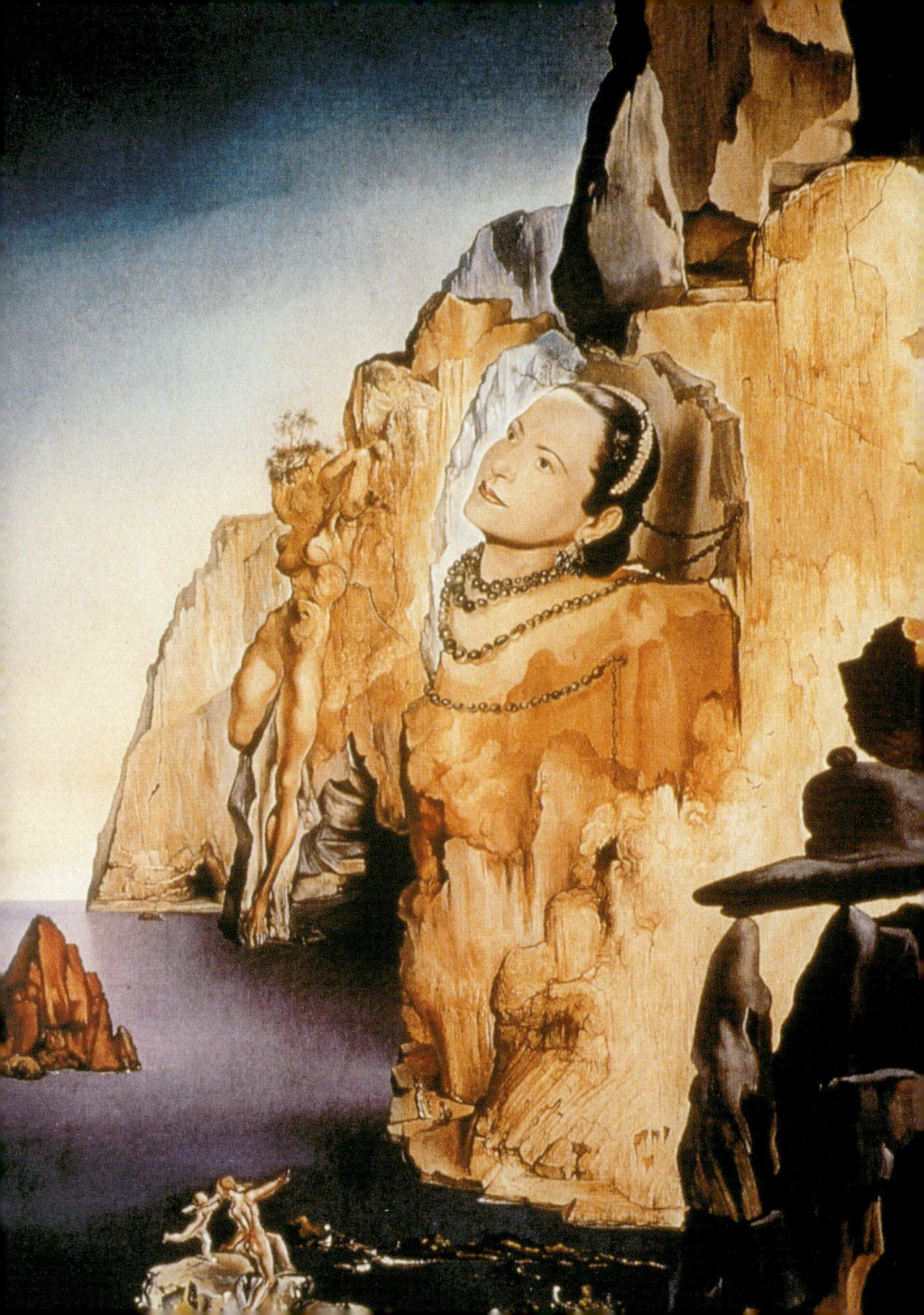

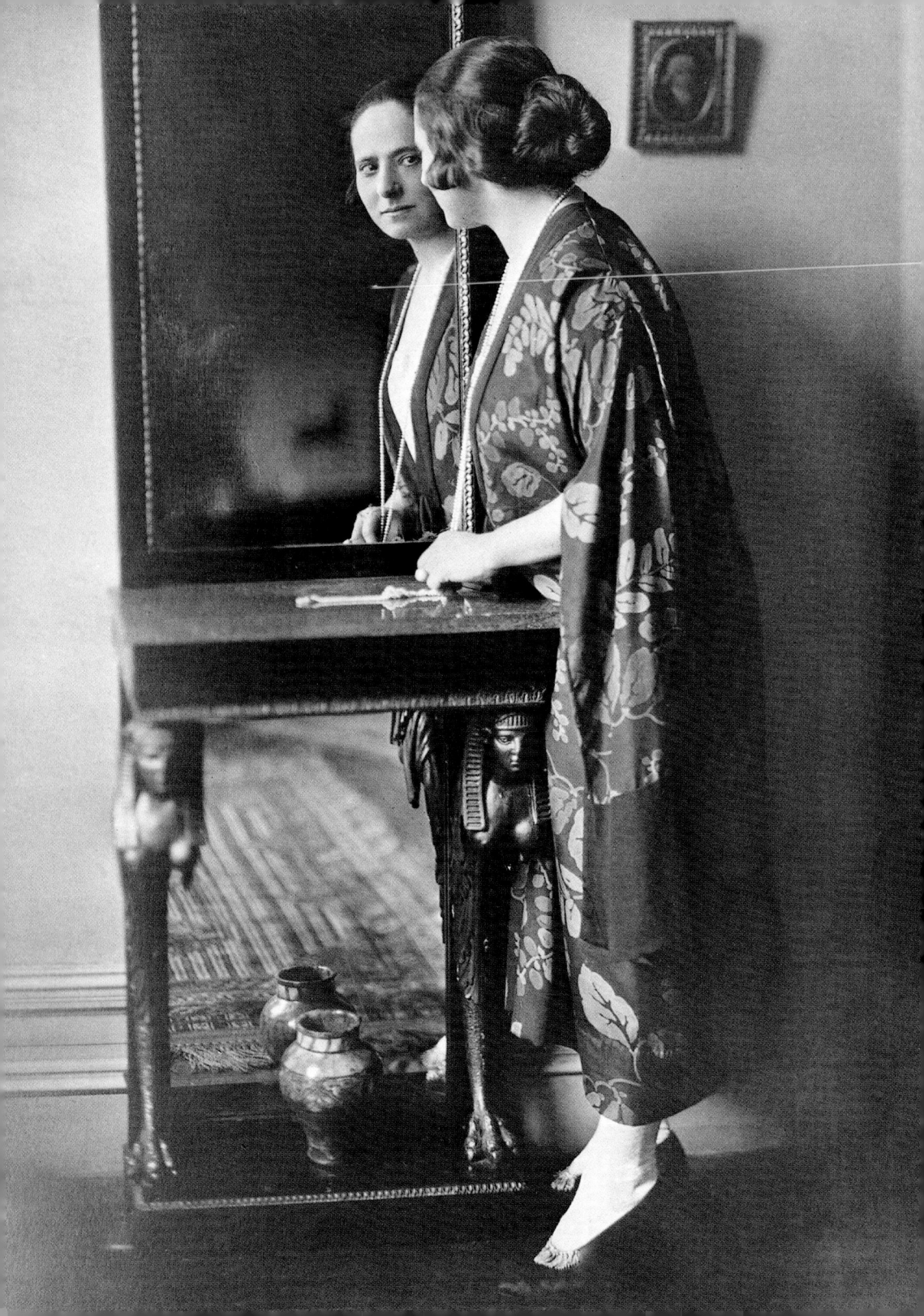

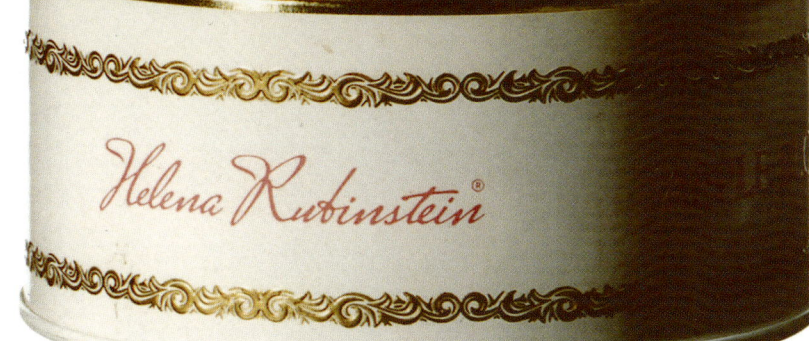

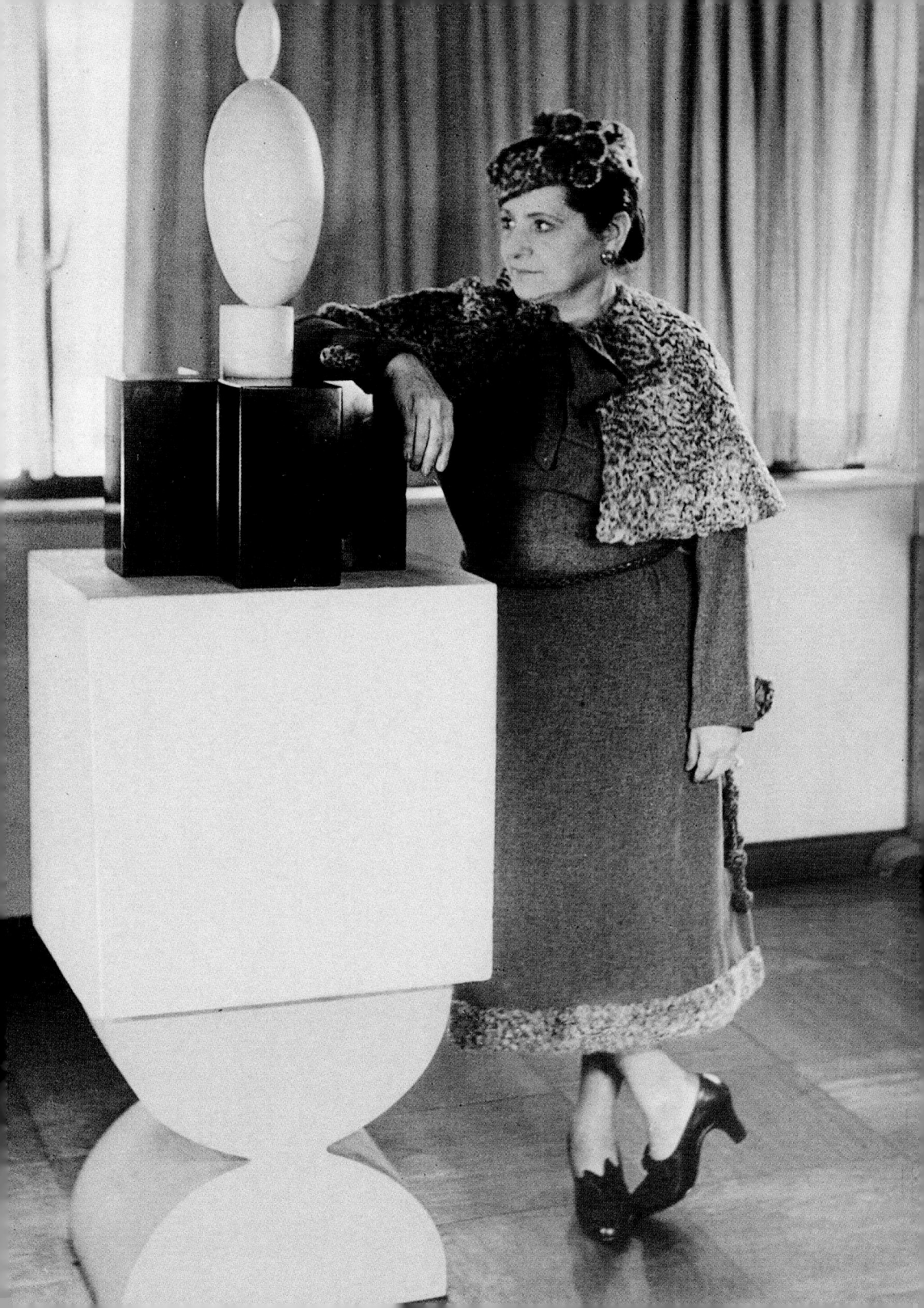

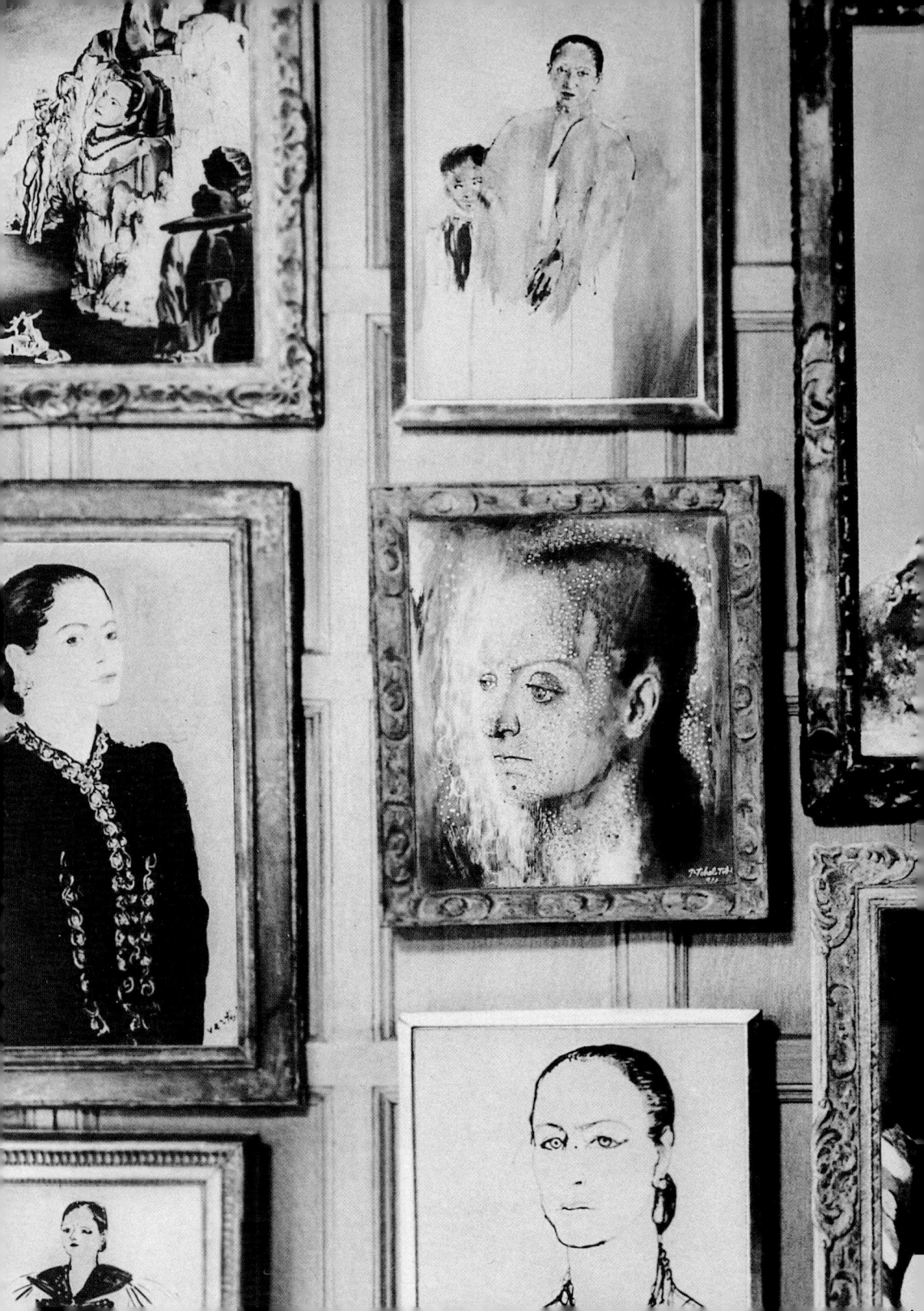

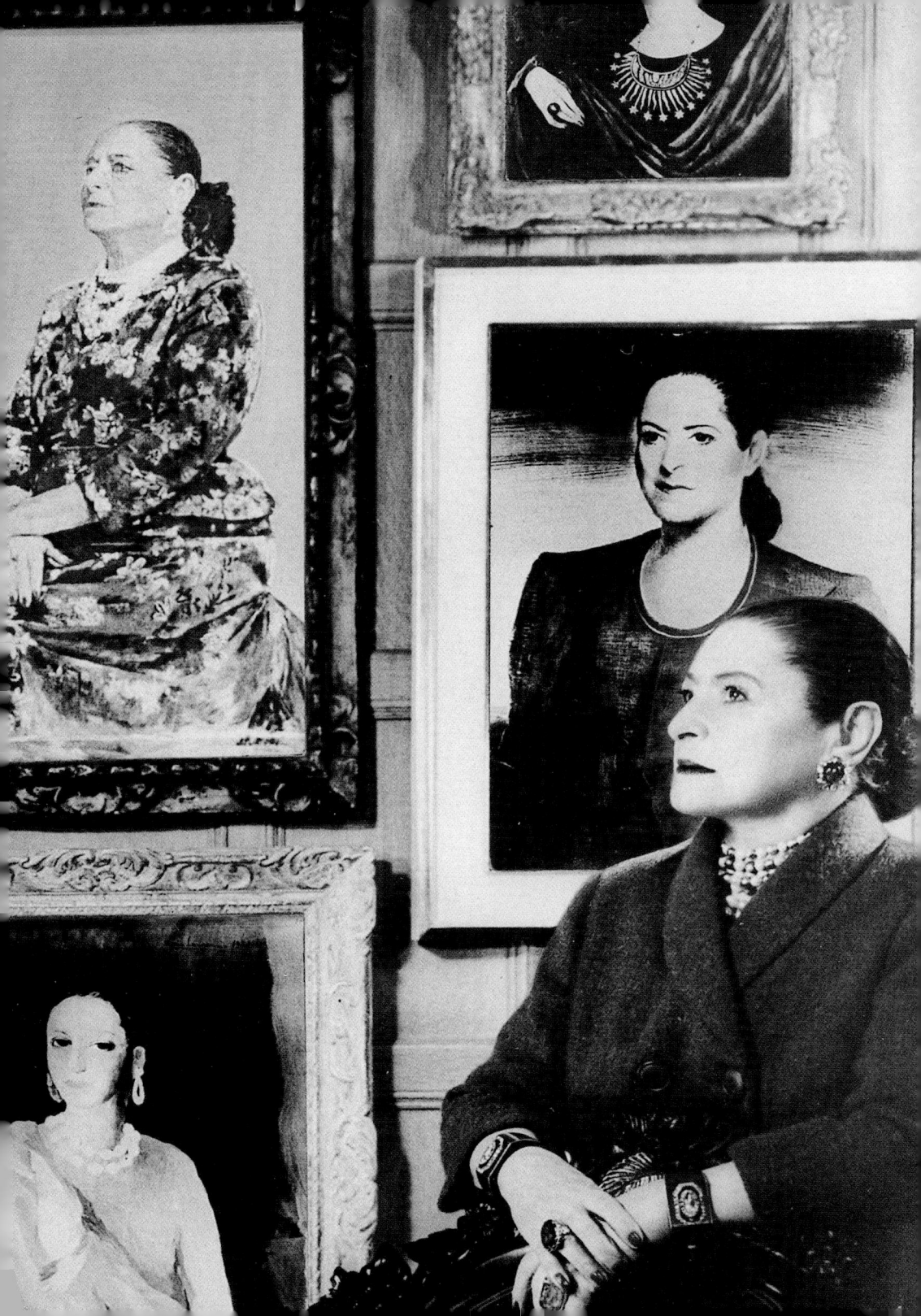

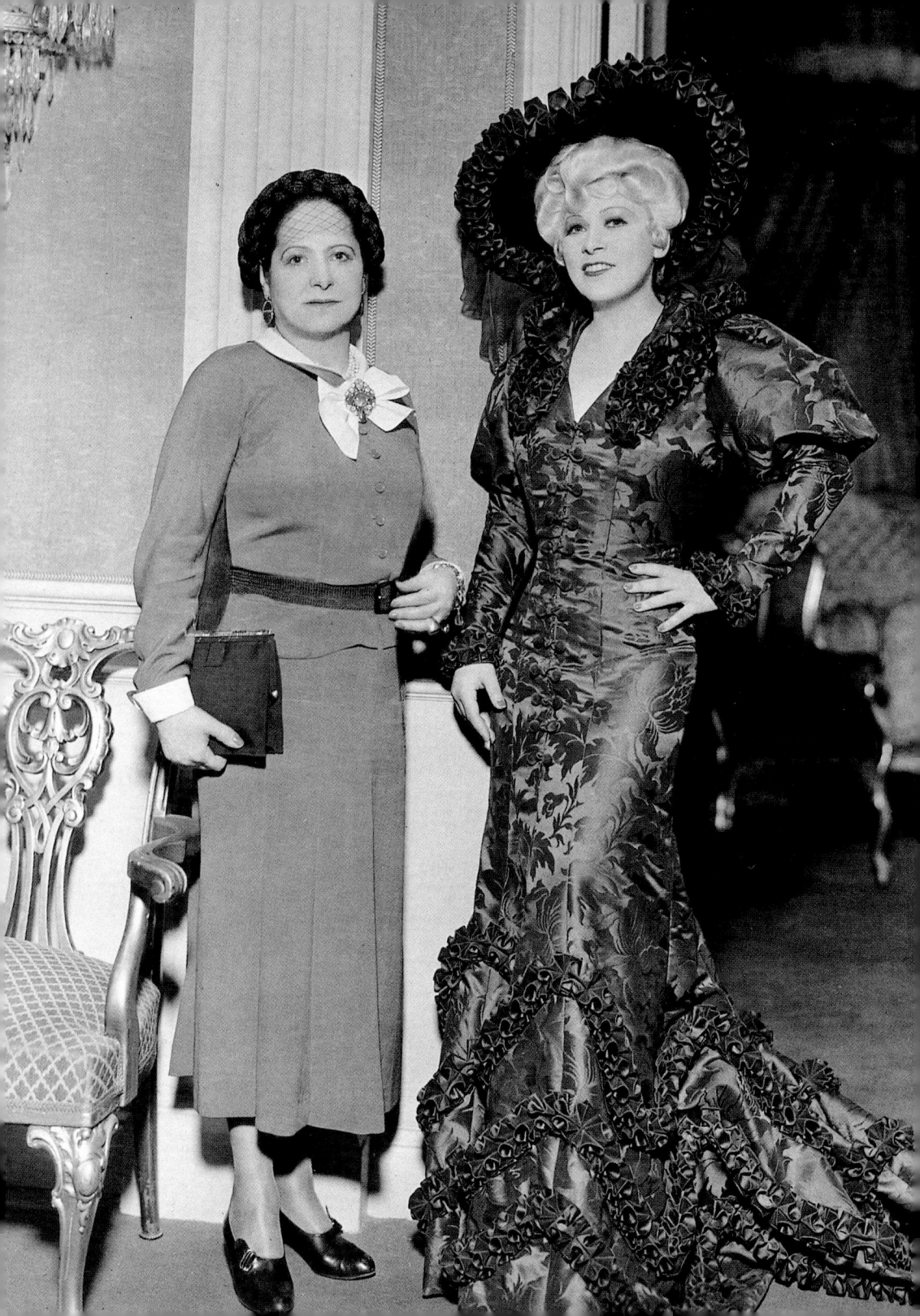

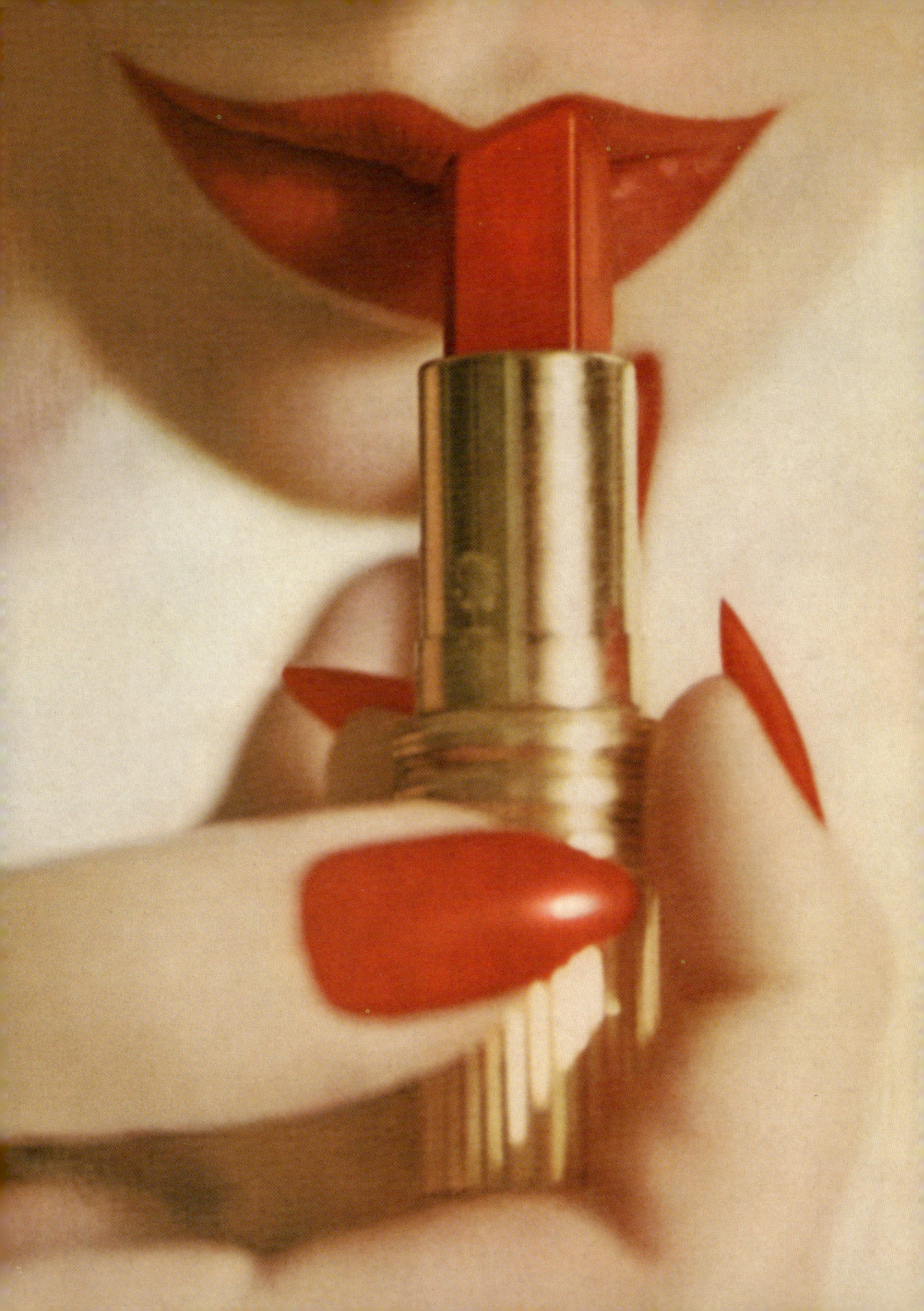

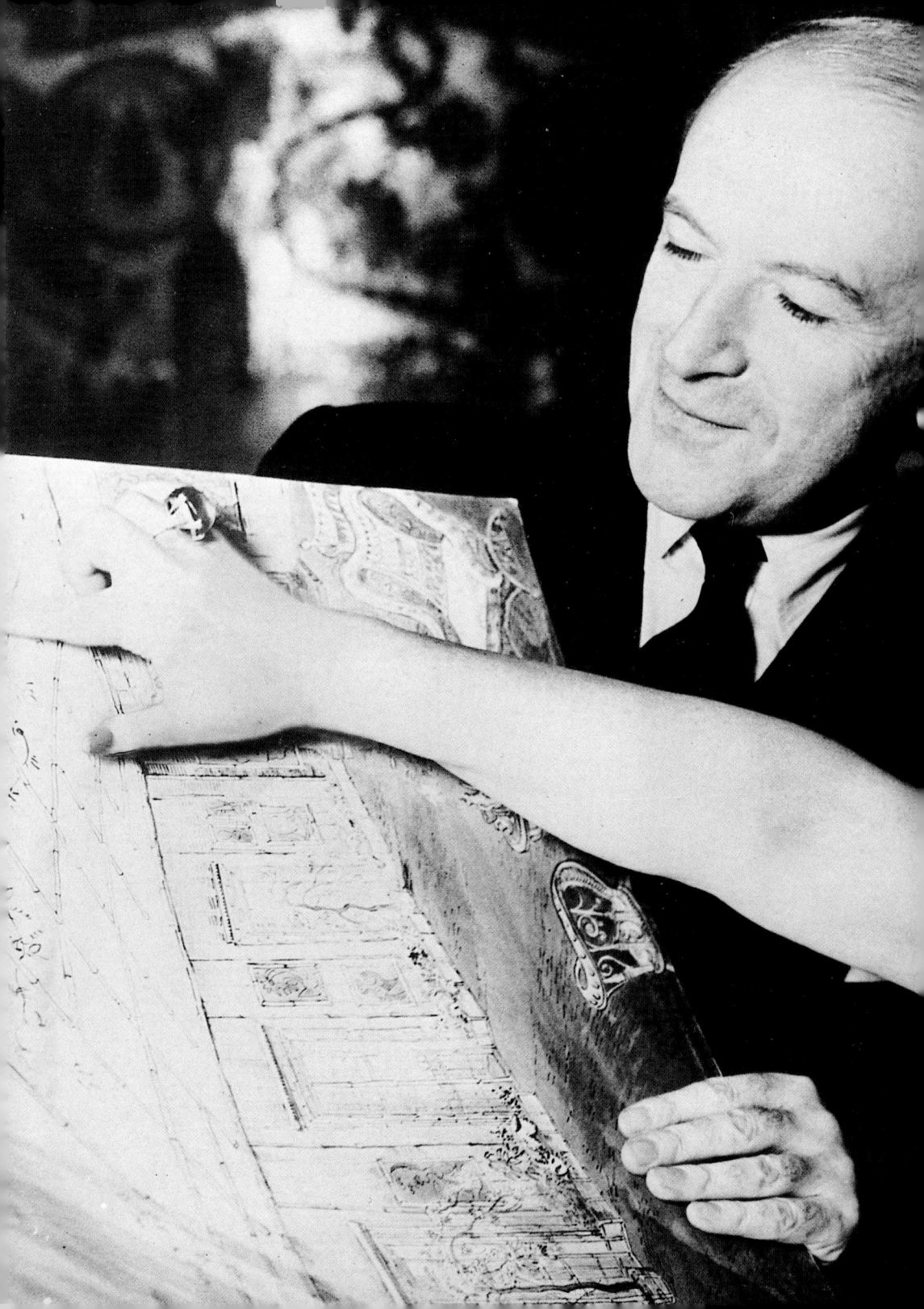

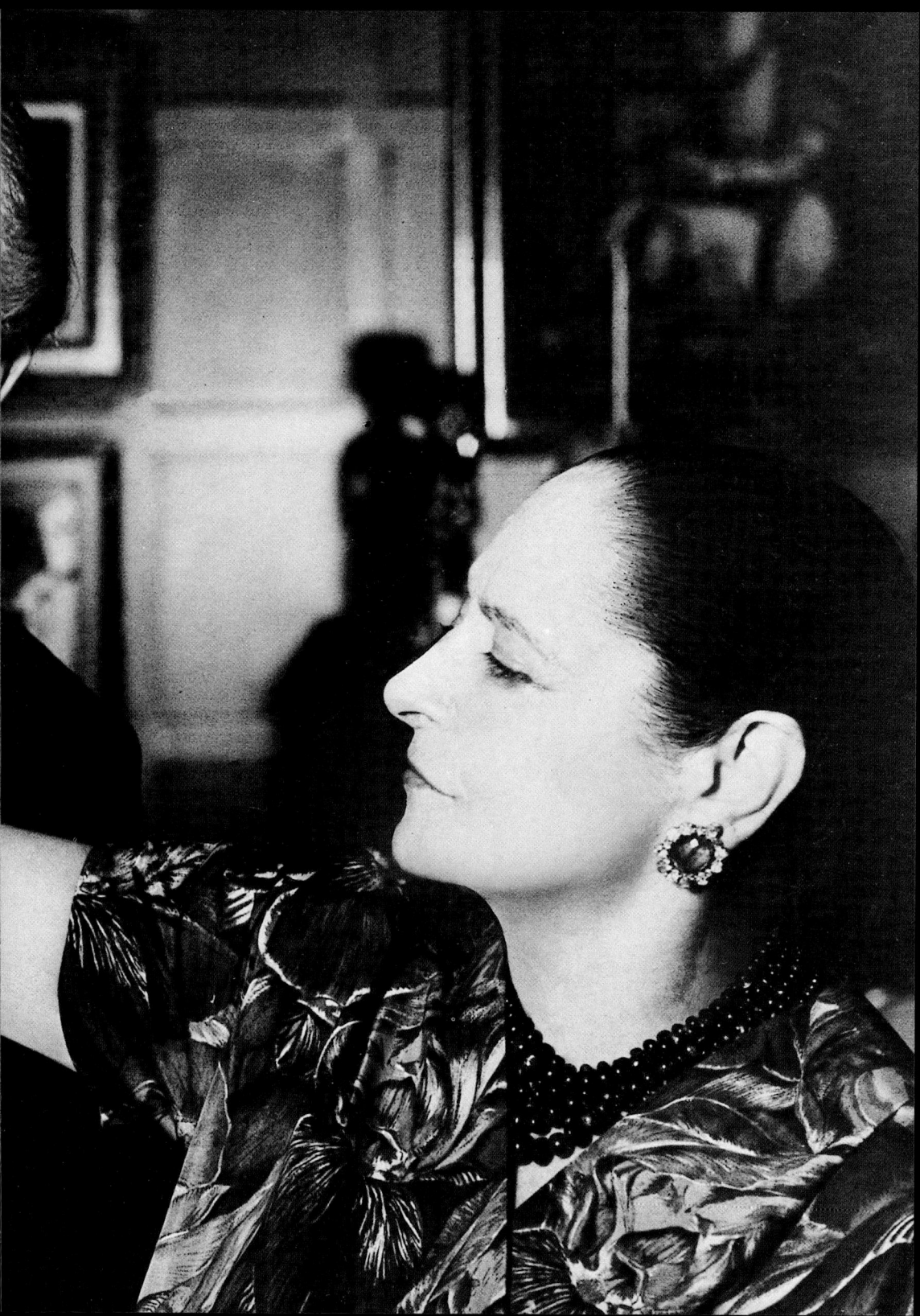

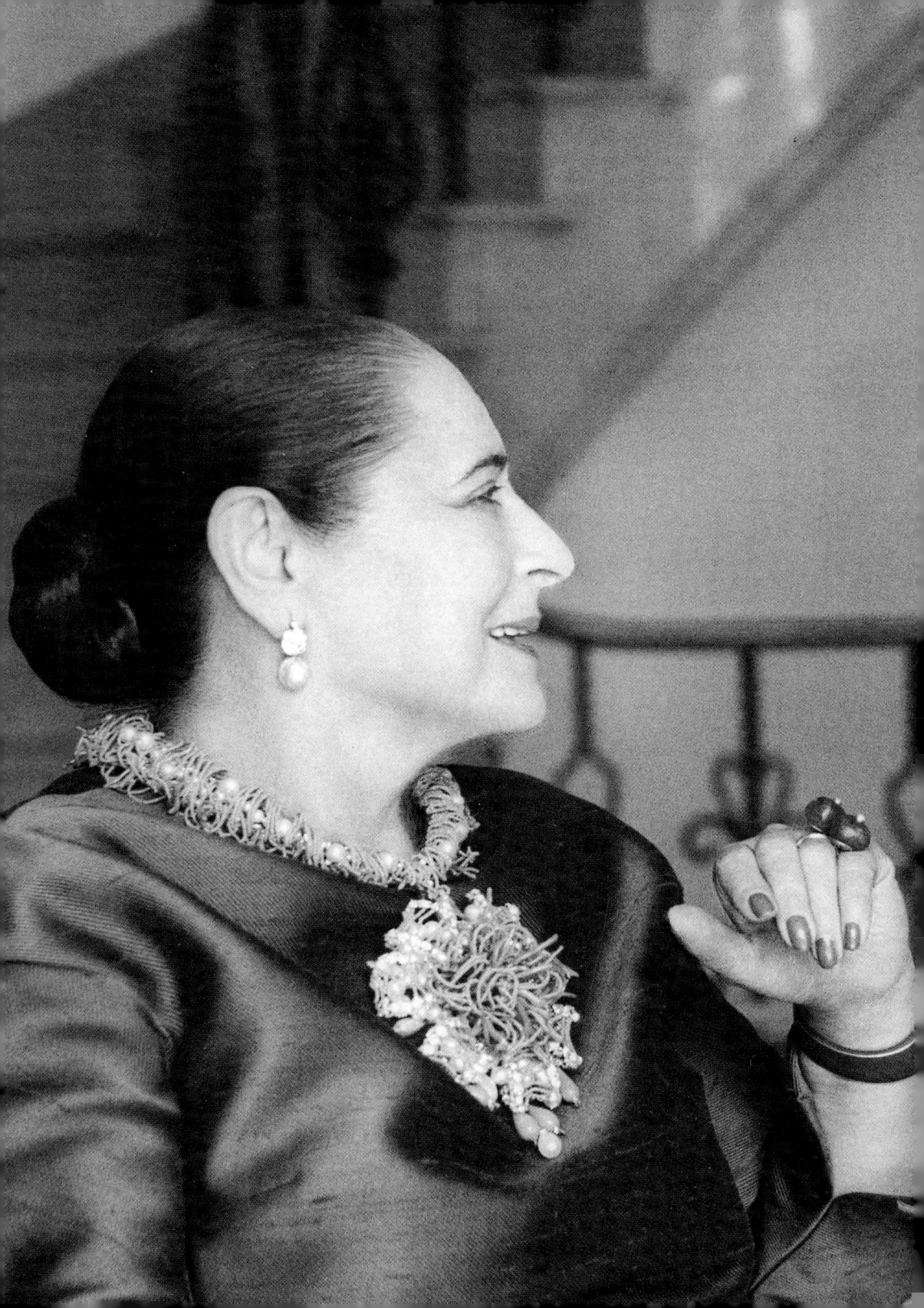

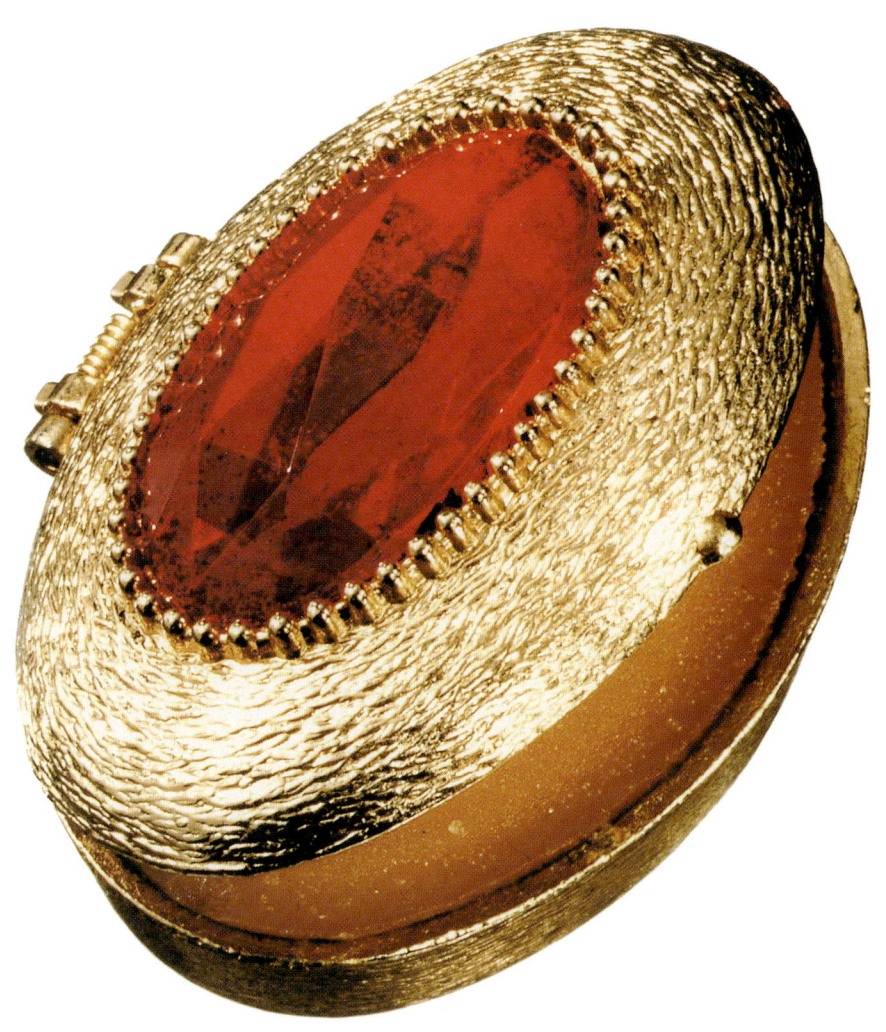

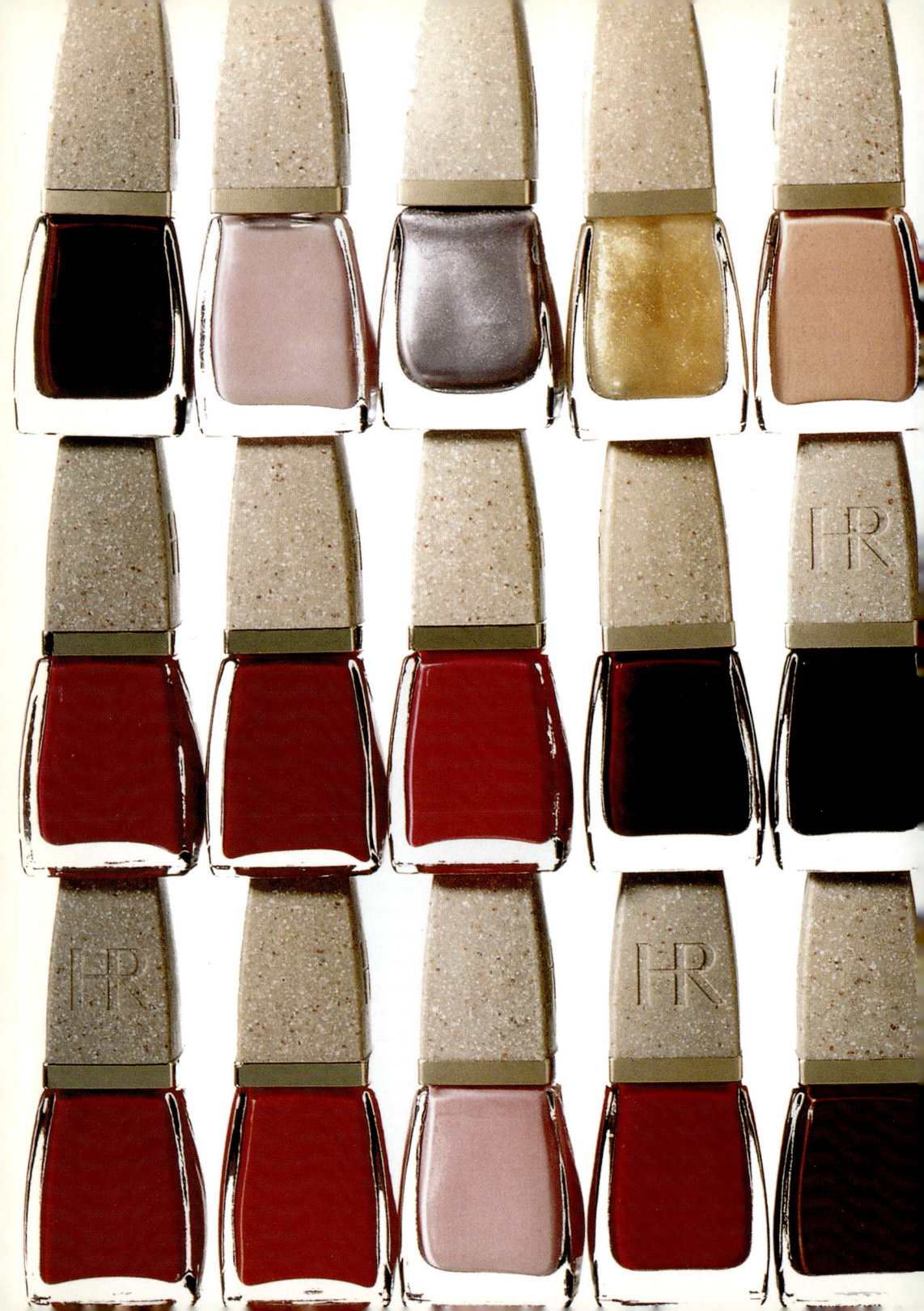

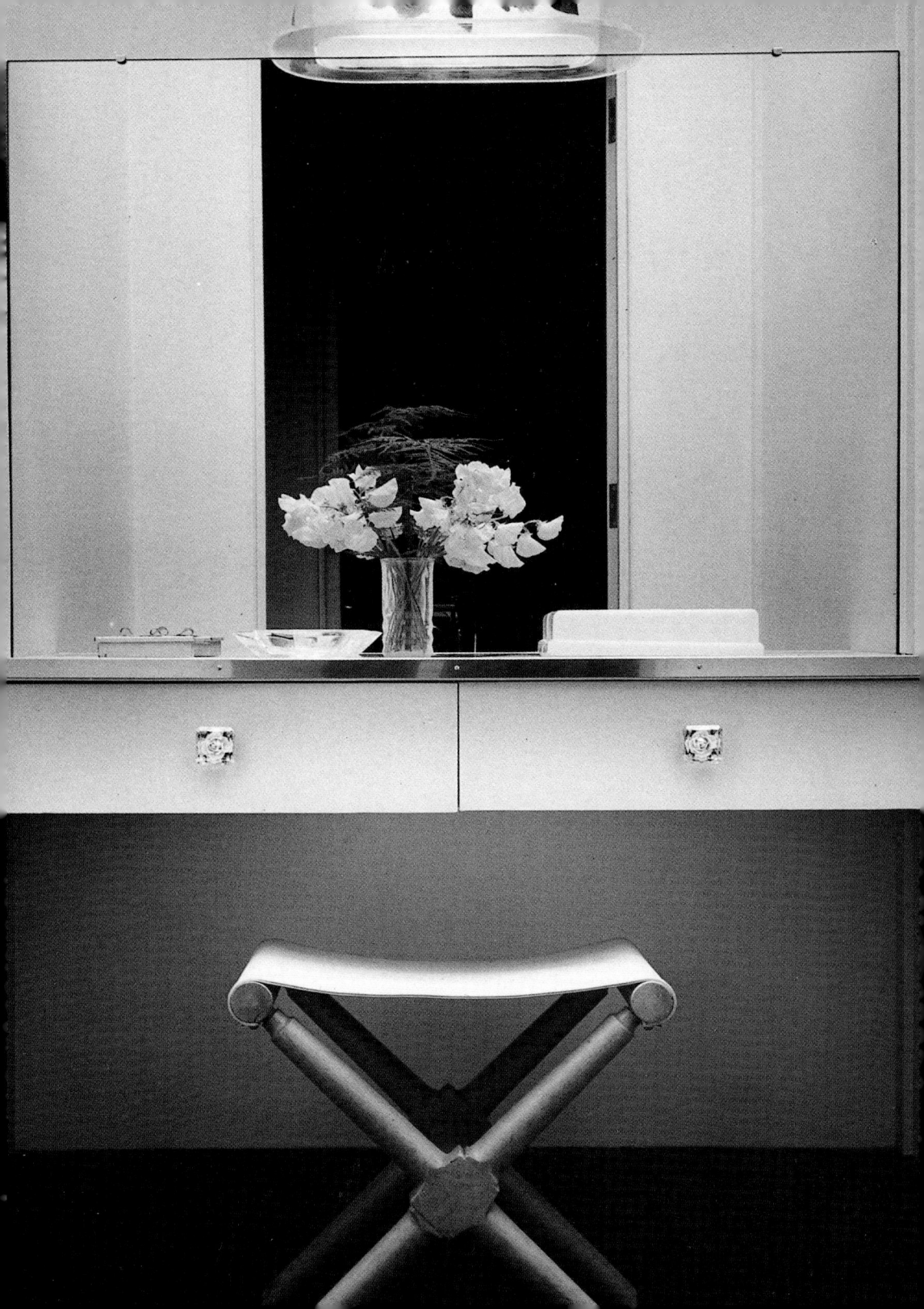

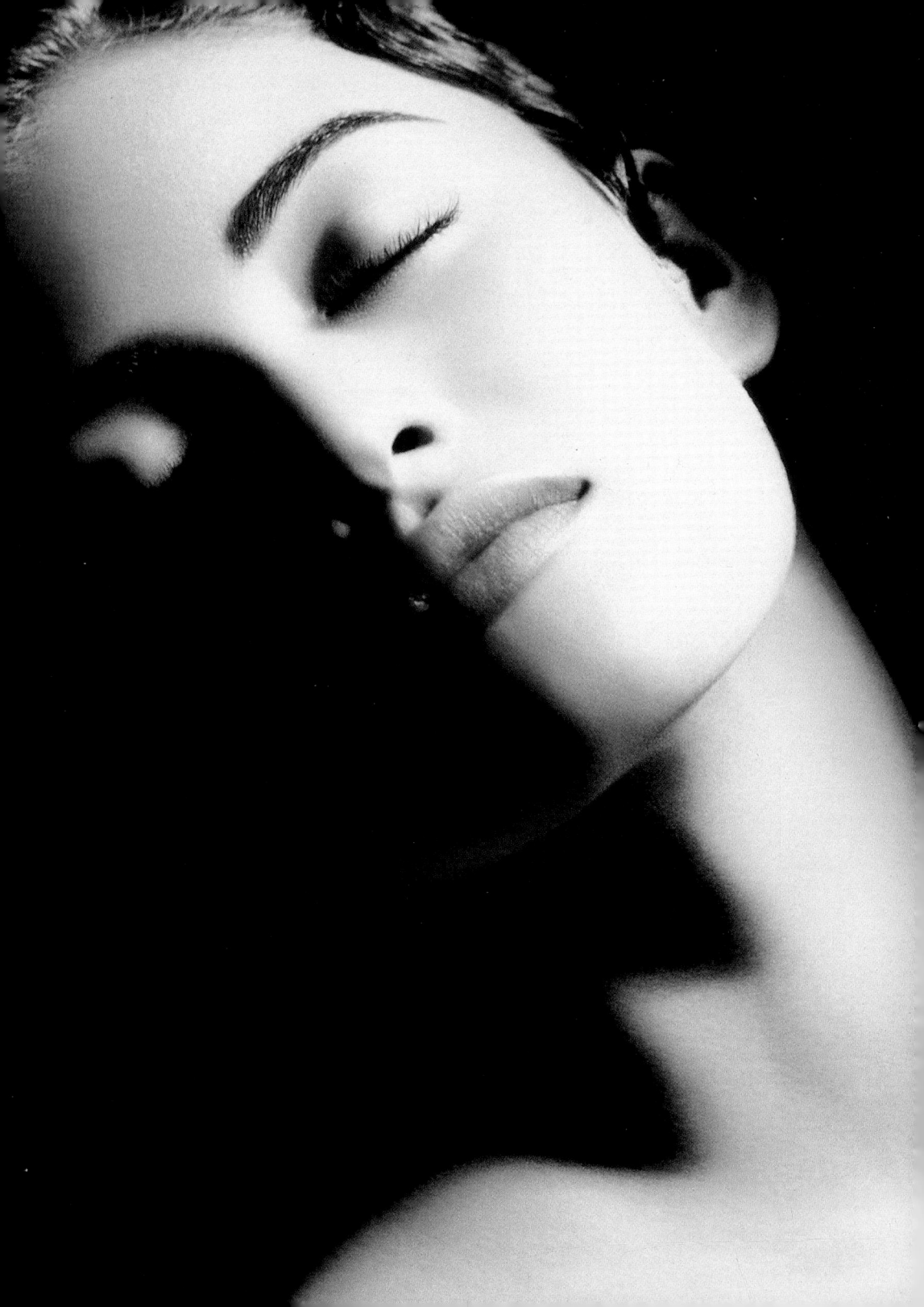

# Chronology

**1872:** Born on 25 December in Cracow, Poland, the oldest of eight daughters.
**1892:** At the age of 20, Helena leaves Poland for Australia, where she stays with a maternal uncle.
**1902:** Inauguration for the *Valaze* beauty salon in Melbourne.
**1905:** Since mail order sales of the *Valaze* cream are constantly increasing, Helena asks the cream's inventor, Dr. Lykusky, to join her and also asks her sister Ceska to come over.
**1905-1907:** Having made her first fortune, Helena hands over responsibility for the beauty salon to her sister and goes on her travels to meet and work with the world's leading skin specialists and dieticians in Berlin, Vienna, London and Paris.
**1907:** She marries Edward Titus in London. He is a journalist of Polish origin, a naturalised American, whom she originally met in Australia.
**1908:** After another short stay in Australia, the Titus family settles in London, where Helena opens the *Valaze* beauty salon at 24, Grafton Street, Mayfair. It is a huge success from the moment it opens.
**1909:** Birth of her first son, Roy.
**1912:** Birth of her second son, Horace.
Opening of the *Valaze* beauty salon in Paris, in the Rue du Faubourg-Saint-Honoré, the city's most fashionable address. Yet again, it is a runaway success.
**1914:** Start of World War I: Helena, her husband and two children leave for New York.
**1915:** Opening of the *Helena Rubinstein* beauty salon in New York.
**1916-1918:** Her fame spreads throughout the United States. Salons are opened in the major cities, such as Chicago and Boston.
At the same time, the *Valaze* beauty care range continues to grow, with new products being added all the time.
**1917:** Helena is persuaded by the most fashionable department stores, the *City of Paris* in San Francisco and *Halle Brothers* in Cleveland, to supply them with her products and to give her consent for direct sales to the public. This will be the start of a new distribution policy for the brand through authorised retail outlets.
**1928:** To everyone's surprise, Helena Rubinstein decides to sell the shares in her American business to the New York bank, Lehman Bros, for the sum of eight million dollars.
She leaves for Europe to join Edward Titus, whom she had never forgotten.
**1929:** After the Wall Street Crash, Helena buys back her company for two million dollars, making a six-million-dollar profit.
**1930:** In Paris, Helena buys an apartment on the Quai de Béthune, on the Ile Saint-Louis, in the middle of the Seine. She commissions Louis Sue, one of the most famous architects of his day, to decorate it. Rubinstein was one of the most sought-after hostesses in Paris between the wars.
**1932:** A *Helena Rubinstein* salon opens in Milan.
**1934:** *Helena Rubinstein* salons open in Vienna and Toronto.
**1936:** Helena Rubinstein and Edward Titus finally divorce.
**1938:** Helena marries the Russian prince Atchil Gourielli, becoming Princess Gourielli.
**1939:** The Acquade Show, a water ballet performed at the New York World's Fair gives Rubinstein the opportunity of presenting a totally new product, the first waterproof mascara, sold over the counter in 1940. It is a huge success worlwide.

*Although a cream cannot replace a face-lift, it can get close to it by using the power of certain ingredients, such as phosphorus.*
*Advertisement for* Face Sculptor, *the first cream to try and reproduce the effects of a face-lift without surgery, 1997.*
© *Photo Christian Moser/Helena Rubinstein Archives.*

**1940:** World War II, and the Gouriellis stay in the United States. throughout the war years, Helena and her family devote themselves to developing the American end of the business.
**1945:** The war is over and Helena returns to Europe. In Paris, the German soldiers have left the salon and offices in the Rue du Faubourg-Saint-Honoré in a dreadful condition. The Grafton Street salon in London has been destroyed by bombs. At the age of seventy-three, Helena decides to rebuild her European empire.
**1950:** Launch of *Deep Cleanser*, a cleansing cream designed to replace *Pasteurized Face Cream*, originally created in the second decade of the century.
**1953:** Introduction of one of the first firming products, *Contour Lift Film*.
**1954:** For the first time in the cosmetics industry, a vitamin-enriched beauty product is created and sold as *Lanolin Vitamin Formula*.
**1955:** Death of Prince Gourielli.
**1956:** *Skin Dew*, the first moisturising skin care product, is launched in June.
**1958:** Launch of *Mascara Matic*, later to become Long Lash. The concept of an automatic refillable mascara was totally new at the time and was received enthusiastically.
**1958-59:** Despite her age (eighty-six), Helena takes a trip to Japan, Hong Kong and Australia. In all these countries she gives countless interviews and lectures, attends events organised in her honour and meets her most important customers.
Three months after her return, Helena leaves for Moscow to attend the American Trade Fair. The U.S. government had asked the firm of Helena Rubinstein to represent the western cosmetics industry at the Fair.
**1965:** On 1 April, Helena Rubinstein dies in her New York home, aged ninety-three.
**1968-1969:** Introduction of *Illumination* to replace *Minute Make-Up*.
**1974:** Helena Rubinstein's heirs sell the company to Colgate-Palmolive.
**1977:** *Silk Fashion*, a new line of make-up based on natural silk is launched in April. It is designed to replace *Illumination*.
**1979:** *Golden Beauty* is launched in January. This range of sun-tan products contains an exclusive ingredient called "Premelanine," which accelerates tanning.
**1980:** Colgate-Palmolive sells all its shares in Helena Rubinstein to Albi International. On 1 December, Helena Rubinstein acquires the distribution rights to Armani perfumes.
**1984:** L'Oréal buys the Helena Rubinstein operations in Latin America and Japan.
**1985:** Launch of the first automatic eyeliner, *Perfect Liner*.
**1987:** Introduction of *Performance H20* in March. The aim is to regain the market share in moisturisers which was lost when *Skin Dew* ceased to be produced.
*Contact Finish*, a liquid make-up based on bioparticles is launched in September.
**1988:** L'Oréal completes the takeover of the Helena Rubinstein brandname, to cover the whole world.
Launch of *Intercell*, an anti-ageing cream based on the principle of intercellular communication.
**1995:** First skin-care product using pure vitamin C.
**1997:** Launch of *Face Sculptor*, containing pro-phosphor.
**1998:** World launch of the *Power A* cream.

*Powder compacts* Silk Fashion Mauresque *(1960s).*
© *Photo Laziz Hamani/Éditions Assouline.*

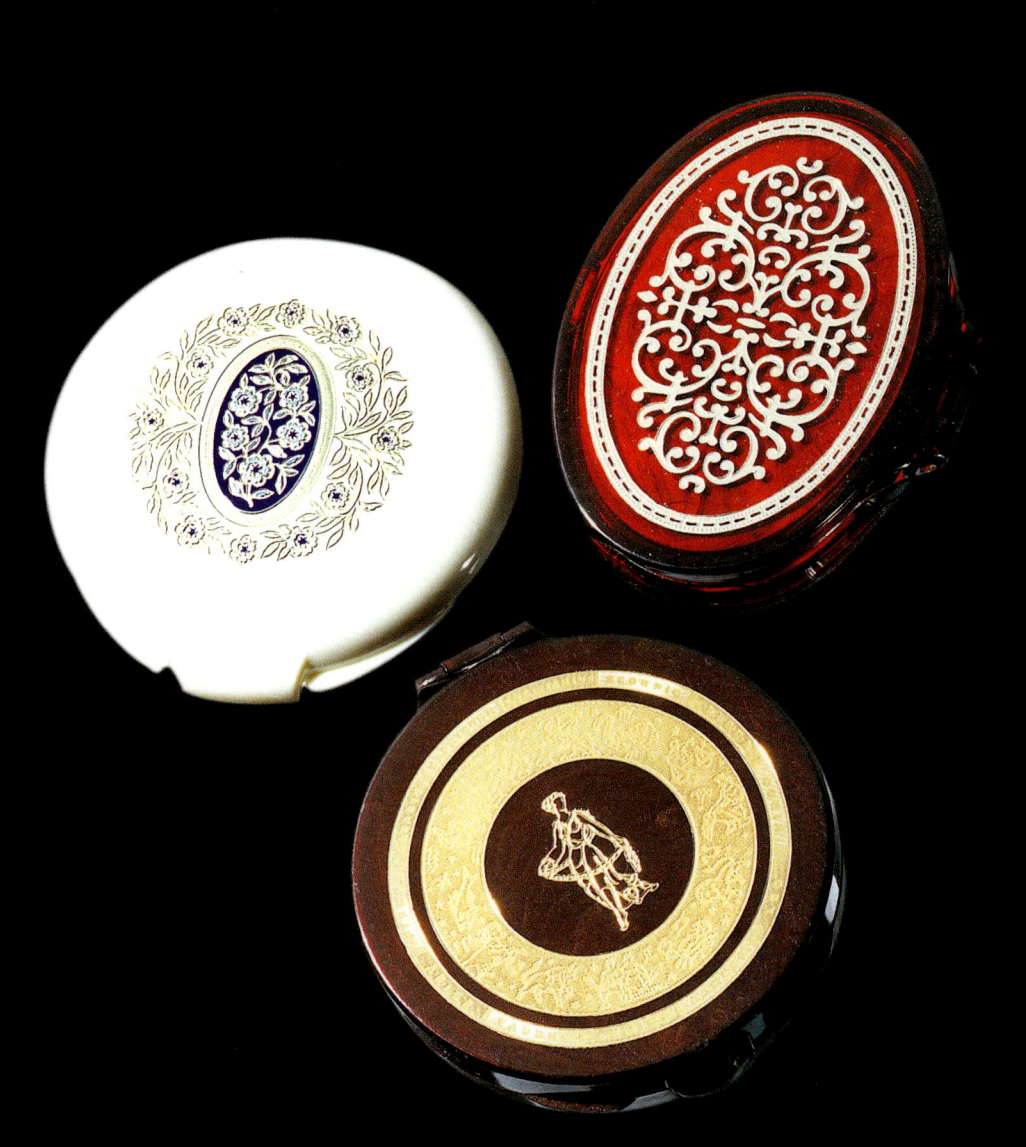

# Helena Rubinstein

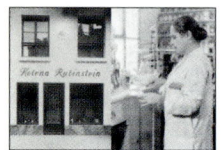

L'Institut de Beauté Helena Rubinstein, 128, Rue du faubourg-Saint-Honoré. © All rights reserved/Helena Rubinstein Archives.
Helena Rubinstein in 1932 in her Parisian laboratory. "I like nothing better than working in my kitchen," she used to say. © All rights reserved/Helena Rubinstein Archives.

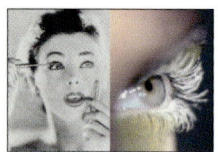

Advertisement for *Silk Fashion,* the first conditioning mascara on the market. © All rights reserved/Helena Rubinstein Archives.
*Dracula,* spring-summer make-up collection, 1998. Art director: Carlos Villalon. © Photo: Christian Moser.

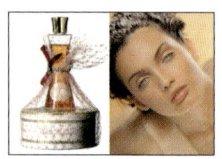

*Dusting Powder* and *Apple Blossom* perfume (1950s). © Photo: Laziz Hamani/Éditions Assouline.
Publicity campaign for *Spectacular Make Up* mascara, 1998. Art director: Carlos Villalon. © Photo: Christian Mosser/Helena Rubinstein Archives.

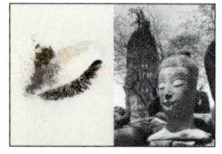

"Make-up is a spectacular mask whose only aim is love. One puts on make-up in order to be looked at, desired, caressed." Left: *Special Effects,* make-up collection, 1996. Art director: Carlos Villalon. © Photo: Christian Mosser (left). © All rights reserved/Helena Rubinstein Archives (right).

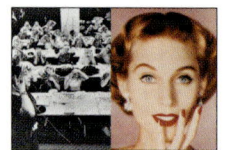

"Beauty is single and indivisible. It is inseparable from the concept of goodness and consequently of happiness." Left: Mala Rubinstein, Helena Rubinstein's niece, training beauticians in massage techniques (New York, 1930s). © All rights reserved/Helena Rubinstein Archives.

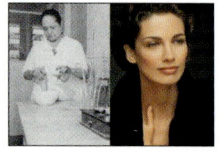

By creating beauty care products which were quasi-medical, Helena Rubinstein showed that beauty was not mere frivolity but a true science. Left: in the late 1950s, Helena Rubinstein still carefully supervised the formulation of her creams. © All rights reserved/Helena Rubinstein Archives. Right: advertisement for *R Vincaline,* a lotion created bio-technologically from the seeds of the Madagascar periwinkle. © Photo: Denis Piel.

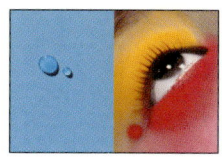

**An emotional approach to colour** by Carlos Villalon, art director for the brand since 1995. © Photo: Jacques-Yves Gucia (left). © Photo: Christian Moser (right).

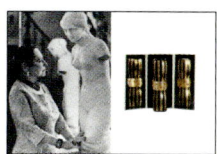

**Everything beautiful fascinates her.** Her taste is eclectic, her apartments nothing short of museums. Left: Helena Rubinstein standing in front of a Greek statue, at the entrance to her Parisian home. The glass-and-chrome door designed by Lalique opens on to Louis XVI sideboards, opaline vases and carpets from Samarcand. © All rights reserved/Helena Rubinstein Archives. Right: *Convertible Lipstick Case*, engraved golden and black enamel (United States, 1950s). © Photo: Laziz Hamani/Éditions Assouline.

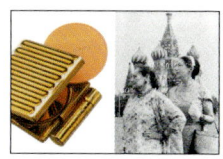

**Lipstick case and powder compact with mirror** (1950s). © Photo: Laziz Hamani/Éditions Assouline.
**Mao in China, Ben Gurion in Israel, Khruschev in the USSR:** on each of her voyages, Helena Rubinstein was received like a world leader. Here she is in 1959, with her niece Mola Rubinstein, in Red Square, at the American Trade Fair in moscow. © All rights reserved/Helena Rubinstein Archives.

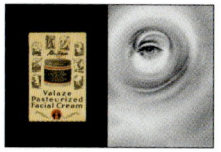

**Leaflet produced in 1905 by her first husband,** Edward Titus, extolling the benefits of *Valaze* cream. Helena Rubinstein had a flair for advertising copy and was often copied by her rivals. © Helena Rubinstein Archives.
**Make-up using** *Silver Smoke Eyeshadow*. Photo by JeanLoup Sieff, published in *Harper's Bazaar*, May 1964. © JeanLoup Sieff.

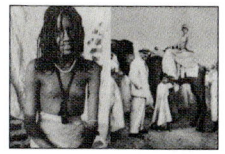

**Impressions of Africa:** on each of her trips, Helena Rubinstein brought back recipes for powders and other preparations which inspired her beauty care products and themes for make-up. Right: Helena Rubinstein and the painter Lurcat on an excursion in Tunisia, 1921. © All rights reserved (left). © All rights reserved (photo: Dorlan)/Helena Rubinstein Archives (right).

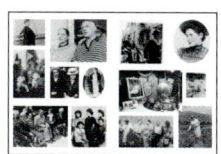

© All rights reserved/Helena Rubinstein Archives.

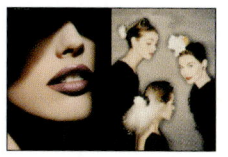

**Institutional image for** *Rouge Glorious* lipstick. Art director: Carlos Villalon. © Photo: Christian Moser/Helena Rubinstein Archives.
**Nancy Berg, Candy Tannev and Elsa Martinelli** wearing dresses by Balenciaga and make-up by Helena Rubinstein. US *Vogue*, October 1954. © Photo: Coffin/1954 by The Condé Nast Publications Ltd.

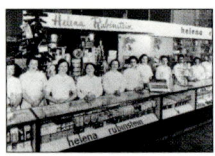
**The Helena Rubinstein display counter in New York department store** in the 1950's. At the time, Helena Rubinstein company was one of the ten biggest cosmetic firms in the United States, with a range of more than five hundred products and a turnover of a million dollar a year. © All rights reserved/Helena Rubinstein Archives.

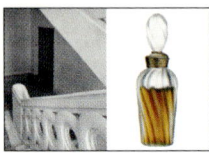
**In 1930s, Helena Rubinstein bought a historic mansion** on the Ile Saint-Louis in Paris from José Maria Sert. The architect Louis Sue was commissioned to convert and renovate it. In 1961, she rented one of the apartments to Georges and Claude Pompidou. © All rights reserved/Helena Rubinstein Archives.
**Flacon of *Heaven Sent* perfume** (United States, 1950s) © Photo: Laziz Hamani/ Éditions Assouline.

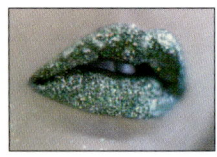
**Non conformity Helena Rubinstein style.** After successfully introducing yellow and green powder and blue and black lipstick, under the influence of the Chilean painter Carlos Villalon, art director since 1995, the brand created sparkle lipsticks in meteorite colors. Shown here, Cinderella, on autumn winter make-up collection, 1998. © Photo: Christian Moser.

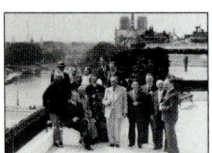
**Occupation: philantropist.** Throughout her life, Helena Rubinstein supported the work of artists. Here she is, in 1953, awarding the Helena Rubinstein Prize, worth twenty five thousand francs to the sculptor Henri Laurens. The jury that year consisted of Henri Matisse, George Braque, Fernand Léger, Louis Marcoussis, Maurice Reynal, Paul Éluard, Henri Laugier, M. Dzarrois, Georges Henri Rivière, Jean Cassou, Mme Cuttou and M. Zervos. © All rights reserved/Helena Rubinstein Archives.

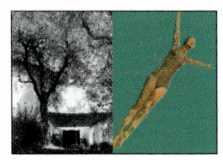
**The White House.** Helena Rubinstein bilt a Moroccan inspired white-and-green house on the hills overlooking Grasse. She also owned the Moulin de Breuil, at Combs-la-Ville. © All rights reserved/Helena Rubinstein Archives.
**Naiade** (May, 1960). © All rights reserved/Helena Rubinstein Archives.

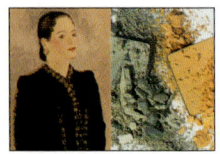
**Portrait of Helena Rubinstein,** dressed in a Balenciaga creation, painted by Paul Vertes in the 1940s. © All rights reserved.
**Creating make-up with the same excitement and the same precision** with which a painter creates a painting. Here: eye shadow from the *Color Choc* collection, spring summer. © Photo: Christian Moser.

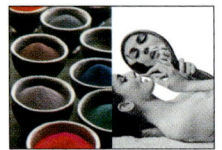
**Painting a face like a picture.** Helena Rubinstein, mother of pearl pigments. The photo appeared in *Elle*, 26 August, 1996. © Photo: Fabrice Bouquet/Elle/Scoop.
**Sun make-up *Bikini Tones*.** *Harper's Bazaar*, July 1965. © All rights reserved/ Helena Rubinstein Archives.

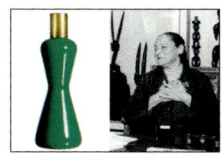

*White Magnolia* **perfume,** 1954. © Photo: Laziz Hamani/Éditions Assouline.
**Helena Rubinstein in her African drawing-room,** Quai de Béthune, on the Ile Saint-Louis. This room, decorated inred and sand, contained a collection of several hundred sculptures of which the most handsome came from Benin. © All rights reserved/Helena Rubinstein Archives.

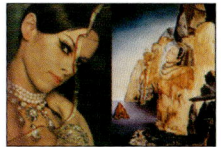

**Geraldine Chaplin** in oriental make-up (1960). Photo: Saul Leiter. © All rights reserved.
**Portrait of Helena Rubinstein by Salvador Dali,** New York, 1942. © Adagp, Paris 1998.

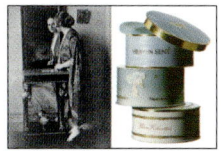

**La Belle Époque:** Helena Rubinstein considered that the years she spent in Paris before World War I, with her husband and sons, were the happiest in her life. Here she is photographed in 1913, in Paris, in a kimono designed by Paul Poiret. © All rights reserved/Helena Rubinstein Archives.
***Apple Blossom* and *Heaven Sent* scented powders** created between 1957 and 1961. © Photo: Laziz Hamani/Éditions Assouline.

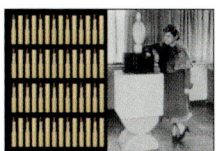

*Spectacular Rouge*, a stay-put lipstick launched in 1996. © Photo: Laziz Hamani/ Éditions Assouline.
**In 1936, Helena Rubinstein purchased *Négresse blanche* by Brancusi.** She is wearing a Molyneux suit. © All rights reserved/Helena Rubinstein Archives.

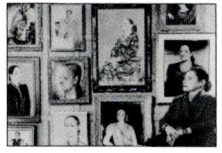

**Helena Rubinstein posing in front of the portraits** her friends painted of her. They include Dali, Vertes, Laurencin, Dufy, Sutherland, Tchelitchev, Portinari. © All rights reserved/Helena Rubinstein Archives.

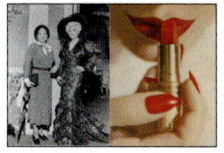

**With Mae West** in 1910. © All rights reserved/Helena Rubinstein Archives.
**The actress Kay Kendall advertising** *Heart of Red* lipstick (1959). © All rights reserved/Helena Rubinstein Archives.

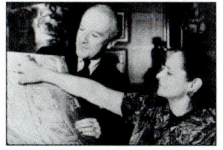

**In Spring 1959, Helena Rubinstein commissioned Sir Cecil Beaton** to decorate the picture gallery in her apartment on Park Avenue, New York, in Japanese style. The walls were lined with bamboo, the ceiling evoked the sky seen through a trellis, and the furnishings were Victorian. © All rights reserved/Helena Rubinstein Archives.

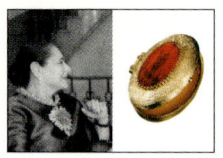

**Helena Rubinstein was inspired by jewellery** in designing her powder compacts and lipstick cases. Paris, June 1962. © All rights reserved/Helena Rubinstein Archives.
*Heaven Sent Perfume Compact,* 1950-1955. © Photo Laziz Hamani/Éditions Assouline.

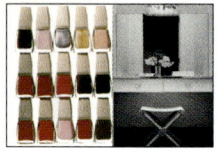

Helena Rubinstein *Nail Lacquer.* © Photo Laziz Hamani/Éditions Assouline.
**Dressing-room of the Helena Rubinstein Beauty Salon** in New York. © All rights reserved/Helena Rubinstein Archives.

The publisher would like to thank the Helena Rubinstein company, and especially Béatrice Dautresme, Anne Cohade and Elizabeth de Hennezel for the help they have provided in the creation of this book.
Thanks are also due to Fabrice Bouquet, Jacques-Yves Gucia, Laziz Hamani, Christian Moser, Denis Piel and JeanLoup Sieff.
Finally, this book would not have been possible without the contribution of David Abel (*Vogue* US), Emmanuelle Montet (Musée de la Mode et du Textile, Paris), Nicole Chamson (Adagp, Paris) and Elle-Scoop.